AUTISM: MEET ME WHO I AM

AUTISM: MEET ME WHO I AM

*A contribution toward an educational, sensory,
and nutritional approach to Childhood Autism
that supports families and ignites the child's
deeper wish to connect to people and the world*

Lakshmi Prasanna
&
Michael Kokinos

Lindisfarne Books | 2018

Published by Lindisfarne Books
an imprint of SteinerBooks/Anthroposophic Press
610 Main Street
Great Barrington, Massachusetts 01230

www.steinerbooks.org

   print ISBN: 978-1-58420-936-2
e-book ISBN: 978-1-58420-937-9

❧ CONTENTS ❧

PROLOGUE IN VERSE

A Doctor Meets Autism
by Lakshmi Prasanna

Coming from the world of mainstream trained
neonatal intensive doctors,

where I mastered seeing everything measurable,
tangible,

where I learnt to describe everything I see,

I struggled in meeting children with autism.

I was challenged in my existence as trained physician

Ground under my feet crumbled...

In meeting these children

I saw the world through their eyes

I heard sounds through their ears

I am reborn in that space, between their seeing and
hearing

And found ground under my feet again

I struggle now to describe what I have seen

And to form words out of what I hear

And I struggle with the world which got lost in fast
moving images and

In noise with no intervals…

So after lot of deliberation,

I decided to open my Heart in this book and write in
my style.

This is an attempt to share what I have seen and what
I have heard.

In my words, you might hear me singing what I have
seen

or images out of the music I heard in their silence.

I am still in this journey,

where I travel between two worlds many times in this
book.

I invite You to come with Me, meeting them,

And Me coming back from that meeting,

To meet You all.

INTRODUCTION

"My heart longs to join in thy song,
but vainly struggles for a voice.
I would speak, but speech breaks not into song,
and I cry out baffled. "
      —*Rabindranath Tagore*

"I'm following cosmos and going a fine balance
between here and there.
I'm going to lift the world into fine balance.
History laughs, but I can do it.
My song is that. I'm trying to sing. "
      —*Akshaya, 12 years old, Chennai, India*

This is a book for parents and families, teachers and schools, doctors and therapists searching for a deeper understanding of the child with autism. The children themselves have led us on a pathway through our striving to connect and communicate our efforts to heal and educate them. This book will share that pathway of two-way learning and healing.

Too often, teachers, doctors, and therapists organize themselves separately in professional groups, searching in isolation for a way to help the individual child before them. And with the same aims, parent support and advocacy groups have been formed worldwide. The "autism puzzle" is a great unsolved mystery of our times. With the latest figures as high as 1 in 60 children, there are a staggering number of families affected, many of them lost within the pieces of the puzzle. Many professionals in the field find themselves swimming in a whirl of conflicting information with no clear evidence based outcome measures to guide them. Adding to the confusion, the rapid advances in technological medicine stand lamed when it comes to this mystery. Your doctor cannot order a scan or test and point to a part of the body, blood, or brain saying, "OK, there it is, that explains the behavior." Understanding complex conditions like autism is one of the great challenges to scientific and phenomenological research in our times.

The outlook on autism presented here emerges out of twenty years of clinical work and individual research. Lakshmi is a developmental pediatrician and neonatologist from India. Michael, an Australian physiotherapist specializing in neurology and the relationship of movement and sensation. Our work has taken place mostly in the rapidly developing cities of South India. We both have very different professional and cultural backgrounds, with one raised in the East and the other raised in a Greek family in the modern West.

Autistic characteristics present with an incredible diversity; the consultation room alone does not often suffice to really see and understand the unique riddle of an individual child. Our interest and research has been to observe the children *contextually*—to look behind the diagnostic labels (communication disorder, repetitive behaviors, lack of eye contact, etc.)—while holding questions such as these:

- How does the child's behavior differ at school, at home, at the supermarket, or at meal times?
- Why is this child so different with different people?
- What influence do different types of food have?
- What sensory need lies behind repetitive behaviors?

- How do siblings, grandparents, parents handle the challenges presented by autism—what are their views?

What followed was a period in our research where one or both of us stayed over in the homes of these children. ("Yes, we are coming for a sleepover!") We would say to the surprised parents, "We would like to come and live with you in your home for two or three days. We would like to really observe your child throughout a few days of their life." We are grateful to the families in India and Singapore who said yes to this unusual request and welcomed us into their homes.

Through this approach, our medical questions became also social, pedagogical, and environmental. We have been challenged to step out of our confining professional silos and expand our circles to begin to work together in a dynamic and developing therapeutic community which includes the parents. This book tells the story of this co-working—because the story, the process, and the outcome are all bound together.

Along the way, professional attitudes and approaches needed to become warmed and humanized. In terms of results, there was much failure and exasperation, together with a degree of promise and some stunning successes. As a general rule, rigid myopic viewpoints and heroic solo efforts simply did not work (at least not for long). Always and without exception the children themselves are our guides and teachers.

We have been fortunate to witness and accompany a group of children in India over the last ten years as they grew from childhood into adolescence and adulthood. Some of these children we first met when they were between seven and ten years old and presenting with severe nonverbal autism. Most of the quotes you will read in this book are from these Indian children with a history of severe autism. Gradually we witnessed the unfolding capacity to communicate and write using a computer, a pen, or the spoken word. What emerged from out of their previously mute souls has been a shock and a surprise to us and to those around them.

Outwardly they appeared illiterate, devoid of emotion, aloof to worldly matters, unpredictable, even prone to violent outbursts. *Inwardly*, they have proved to be astoundingly perceptive, intelligent, sensitive, and empathic far beyond what most had expected. These children have demonstrated a capacity to sense and express their ideas regarding the effect of the mood and feelings of the people around them. They also write about their purpose and hopes—their wish to change the world around them. This has informed our research and ideas.

The original impetus for this book emerged from a seminar on autism organized by Gene Gollogly at New York University in March 2017. The inspiration for writing it has come from the children themselves and their messages, their words, and their strong will to communicate with us. At times it was, as Tagore has put it in the above quotation, a "baffled cry," begging for translation. This is one of the key ideas in this book—that behavior is language and these children are relieved when they meet a capable translator. The New York conference was the first occasion we had to present our perspectives along with the words of the children themselves. How stunning and unexpected for us, that the typed words of our nonverbal, severely autistic children, so many thousands of miles away in South India, would resound in a room overlooking the New York City skyline. Those present felt the power of the children's words that weekend, and this book is dedicated to those same children—in service of what they themselves have termed their earthly mission: Operation Love.

"Meet Me Who I Am" is a poem written to his school teacher by Prasaad—a young man with ASD in Chennai, South India.

Meet me in the good times
Meet me in the mad
Meet me where the river parts
Into the rimp of sea

Meet me when I'm distant
Meet me when you're cold
Meet me when the world ends
On our river boat

Meet me when the sun fades
Meet me when I cry
Meet me when tomorrow ends
Into the end of life.

Meet me when I'm dancing
Meet me who I am
Meet me in the space of
Guilt and hope inside

Meet me in our loving
Meet me in our grief
Meet me I'm inside you
Forever, forever to be.

Many researchers have labored to meet the challenges set before us by each child with autism. We wish to acknowledge the work of so many toward an understanding of autism which balances evidence-based materialistic science with an appreciation for the reality of the human soul-spirit, as well as honest enquiry into the meaning of illness. Autism, we feel, by its very nature, transcends a reductionist materialistic view and points toward the working of soul and spirit in the birth and growth of our children. Our intention was always to be guided by the objective facts themselves, and to let these speak to us.

1

OUR STORIES:
THE JOURNEY TO MEET AUTISM

*"I am Sabari, your witness, your watchman, your
biographer and your author.
I plan to write your story, for it is my journey too.
I am your mirror of sun."*
—Sabari, at age 18, letter to Lakshmi, December 2016

LAKSHMI'S STORY

As a young doctor I was employed in public and private hospitals in Chennai and Hyderabad, South India, while taking specialist training in pediatrics and neonatology (newborns). In the city's main intensive care unit, I was disturbed to see children and babies in the same room as adults without specially trained staff.

I held a vision for something better, and in a few years I set up the first private pediatric intensive care unit at CDR Hospital Hyderabad. I trained all the staff myself and we were given a separate unit for children and babies. Later I started my own private hospital called Little Hearts Children's Hospital. As a practicing neonatal intensive care doctor running my tertiary care unit, I was very busy. In addition to twenty beds of neonatal intensive care, there was an outpatient clinic. It was also my home, I lived and worked there.

Little Hearts became known in Hyderabad as a center of excellence for high risk pregnancies and newborn care. I was busy with following up high risk newborns for developmental challenges and working with a team of physiotherapists and trained nurses in developmental assessments and early intervention. We cared for children with cerebral palsy, downs syndrome, speech delay, and ADHD, as well as premature babies and deaf-mute children. I also visited the Spastics Society regularly. Little Hearts also became well known in the city for helping babies and toddlers with developmental delay.

I started seeing more families with children with attention deficit and hyperactivity syndromes. In my practice, I noticed that these children often had associated digestive weakness or intolerance to food or history of speeded-up milestones.

So working with diet protocols eliminating processed food, wheat, and milk became one of the first steps in approaching these children. I suggested a gluten free/casein free diet with the whole family following a new lifestyle wherever possible. I learnt that when the whole family changed their diet patterns and lifestyle with dinner and bedtime before 7 pm, the children showed consistent improvement in attention and behavioral patterns. Some severe ADD/ADHD children became completely better. Of course, some ADHD children did not respond to diet alone.

Around this time, I had my first encounter with autism. What struck me deeply out of this meeting was that I did not seem to exist for this child. There was no differentiation between me, the person, and my stethoscope, as he reached out and pulled the instrument from my neck. It was deeply disturbing for me to meet a child who was not aware of another human being's presence in the room. The sense I had that he could perceive *objects* clearly, but did not seem to perceive *me*, stayed with me for a long time. I had more children like this visiting me in the clinic during the following months, and I started asking questions. I started a new file where I put these children who were difficult to help. Many other centers refused to see them. This journey, which started more than twenty-five years ago, has become my path.

My early years were focused on working with nutritional programs and exploration of all possible ways of cleaning the gut, including antifungal treatments and various supplementation products. Ayurvedic medicine has its origins in South India, and working with and researching in collaboration with traditional Ayurvedic practitioners gave me the possibility to move quickly into holistic, balanced, individually designed programs with the least amount of supplementation products or pharmaceutical, chemically produced medications.

Improvement in sleep and ease in managing children at home through everyday life around basic needs were my early observations with this step in improving gut function.

Simultaneously working with sensory integration programs and the immediate environment of the child at home and school was taken up, and this was the beginning of building therapeutic communities around each child.

Also at this time, I took my first steps into working with Carnatic music, which later became deeply integrated into the special school curriculum with two experienced music therapists employed on staff. I found the children could connect to rhythm and music as a bridge. Carnatic music is an indigenous traditional music with a deep connection to the ancient devotional traditions of Hindu South India. It also has a medical aspect of music therapy as well as an orientation to the natural world—e.g. seasons and day/night cycles. Children who were otherwise unable to follow instructions could sit still and imitate the rhythm by tapping the right hand on the thigh. This is how Carnatic music is traditionally taught—through the rhythm (*Tala*) as primary. There are specific melodies (*Ragas*) directed toward gut cleansing and strengthening.

I also came across the work of Rudolf Steiner at this time—Waldorf education and anthroposophical medicine. Learning and diving simultaneously and deeply into anthroposophy and Ayurveda greatly helped me in this initial part of the journey of understanding children on the spectrum.

We had our first "summer camp" for this batch of kids in 2003–2004. It was a six-week program with a simple curriculum. My daughters were on summer holiday and needed something to do—they became wonderful helpers playing traditional games with these kids. These games involve challenging fine and gross motor skills, attention, and social interaction. The curriculum consisted of: nutrition; traditional Indian games; music.

Mainly I just watched—observing each child keenly. I saw that in these children the senses were not coming together to form a whole picture. This led me to read everything I could find on sensory integration. I travelled to Kerala to meet traditional doctors and learn from them. Ayurvedic texts speak of "eleven senses plus the one." I was curious about this because Rudolf Steiner also speaks of twelve senses. I watched and concluded that each child had a unique set of sensory-motor processing problems.

After the summer camp, many children improved. The parents all said—"we want to stay!" I tried to give them home programs but they wouldn't budge: they wanted a program outside their homes. We had to find a designated space out of which I could continue my work with these children on the spectrum outside my regular neonatal practice and commitments at the Little Hearts Children's Hospital. That is when I started Saandeepani Centre for Healing and Curative Education in collaboration with my colleague Dr. Swapna Narendra. The founding staff members included physiotherapists Sridhar and Sushmitha Reddy.

The birth of Saandeepani

I chose the name Saandeepani out of my encounters and experiences working with these children. The name comes from Hindu mythology. I had these questions in the first few years of meeting children on the spectrum.

- Who is teaching whom?
- Are these children giving us an opportunity to respond to our inner calling?
- Are we educating them? If so, in what?

Around that same time, I heard a story from a friend of mine who is a great scholar in Vedic knowledge:

Saandeepani was a very, very old man who lived at the time when Krishna was born and raised on earth as the eighth incarnation of the god Vishnu. Krishna became famous for his qualities of compassion, tenderness, and love and is one of the most popular and widely revered among Indian divinities. Krishna is the bearer of all knowledge and grew up to be the wondrous guide of the noble and striving bowman Arjuna in the Hindu epic the Mahabarata.

Saandeepani was a teacher. At the end of his life he taught the young boy Krishna.

In the story, the seven-year-old Krishna tells his mother, "There is a teacher for me, his name is Saandeepani, please take me to him." When they arrived, the old man rose up to greet him saying " Krishna, I have been waiting for you. If I can be your teacher this will be my final activity in this life. It is my destiny to be your teacher. This will release my spirit form the earth."

Traditionally, the teacher occupied a plinth and the student sat on the ground. But Saandeepani and Krishna both sat on the same platform. It is said that people who watched then wondered "who is teaching whom?"

Is Saandeepani teaching Krishna? Or is Krishna giving an opportunity for the teacher to fulfill his destiny?

Working with this first group of children with autism in South India, a few of us carried this same question: Are we teaching them? Or are we finding our destiny purpose in meeting them and serving their needs? That is how the name Saandeepani came to us.

Saandeepani located itself in a little house near the Little Hearts Hospital in the year 2004. On the staff, in addition to the medical team, were a dedicated cook and two untrained teachers who were drawn to the children.

Working with parents and families

"Since we cannot change reality, let us change the eyes which see reality."
—*Nikos Kazantzakis, Report to Greco*

At Saandeepani, I worked with changes in lifestyle, deciding food programs, and changes in home environment to suit individual children's sensory needs. This required spending many hours with parents and sometimes with grandparents. In some situations this also involved working with siblings. In most situations, the primary caregiver was the mother, but we also had fathers taking the role of active primary caregiver.

We offered parent workshops about diet and the healthy development of children and its close relation to sensory environment. During these sessions we also explored child development through the inner sensory experience of the child, especially around speech, hyperactivity, and the unusual behaviors we see in these children. We realized that many parents experienced a kind of self-healing by attending.

There were workshops where parents were taken through a journey of exploring the sense of touch and learning basic massage techniques. This empowered many parents in putting children to bed or handling meltdowns at home.

Handwork and craft groups with parents helped to carry certain therapeutic sensory activities into home life. Many families had outdoor and indoor play areas designed to support their child's sensory needs. Swings and rocking chairs helped children with vestibular symptoms. The music therapists worked with individual parents giving very specific exercises to each child and teaching the parents.

Some parents could see the child in a new way by seeing them through my eyes. I would ask the parents to write a description of their child before the first interview. What the parent wrote about the child initially, and what I described after the first meeting was often very different. We spent time and tried to understanding each other and what we were seeing. This helped in building a warm relationship between parent and child and also shifted how the parent experienced this child.

This reduced parental anxiety around behavioral issues and led to more openness and warm interest in working with the child at home. In some situations mothers found the serenity to continue with their life and career paths. Other parents found meaning in reaching out to other parents who are in need. We saw parents starting new initiatives to help more children, becoming special educators, training to become therapists, helpers, and assistants.

Siblings were always part of the picture at Saandeepani. Also, new babies came into these families making a big difference in family dynamics. For parents it was a positive, warm experience to witness what we call normal child development. It was reassuring, freeing from guilt, and also this helped in respecting the child with autism for his or her own way of living.

The relationship between the child on the spectrum and their sibling was special, and on many occasions we experienced big leap of positive development. Later, as the younger children grew up, what was fascinating was how they experienced and described their autistic siblings. There were situations where siblings needed special time and space where they could express their feelings. Once a year we celebrated "Siblings Day," creating a special day for them. Where appropriate, we involved brothers and sisters in practical educational and therapy activities.

The initial work at Saandeepani was guided by the warm collaboration between doctors, therapists, and parents. There was an atmosphere of exploration. Initially, we developed a parent education program, which evolved out of the requests of parents who wanted to learn more about child development, food, behavior and sensory processing in order to help their own children with autism. Some of the parents who took these courses began working at Saandeepani, some went on to study special education and became teachers. The case study here indicates a typical case in South India.

SAI KEERTHANA: THE GOD-GIVEN GIFT

Keerthana…our second child and the only daughter in our family, was born after a gap of eight years following the birth of our son Kalyan. Her mother was very confident that she was going to give birth to a female child. Keerthana's mother spent all the nine months of pregnancy reading holy books and listening to classical music. Hence, we dreamt that the child would definitely flourish in dance and music.

It was on March 12, 2000, at 8:44 pm, the happiest moment—when her mother gave birth to Keerthana. Keerthana was very fair with a birth weight of 3.5 kg. It was a normal delivery. After listening to the baby's cry, my wife asked the doctor "Is that a baby girl?" The doctor replied, "Yes, it is a very beautiful baby girl." We celebrated the day as never before. It was the first baby held and kissed by her brother Kalyan. The very next day, I was promoted to Officer's cadre in my organization. Keerthana is a gift to us.

After her naming ceremony on the twenty-first day, I was transferred to New Delhi. Those were the days, we enjoyed every moment of Keerthana. Her first smile, rolling, crawling, her little words, sitting, first tooth, and her footsteps in the eleventh month and walking—we celebrated every moment. Kalyan enjoyed all his past thru Keerthana's moments. On her first birthday, she welcomed each and every guest. She danced to the music with other kids. She used to run from the kitchen to the TV room, when she heard the songs, ads, and title music of the daily serials. The timely vaccination was done for Keerthana. She used to imitate her mother in sweeping, mopping, and cleaning the household. She used to play with her peer group in the evenings. At twenty months of age, she started crying for a long time in frequent intervals. She stopped paying attention to us and also reduced eye contact. She loved to be alone. There was no improvement in her speech. She used to say only "Amma and Ammamma." She cried twelve to fifteen hours a day. She could not sleep in the night and used to sleep for just two to three hours in the early morning. She was restless throughout the day. It was a big confusion for us, what was happening to our loving child.

We immediately consulted an ENT specialist referred by Keerthana's doctor. The specialist did Audiometry for her and found no fault in her hearing. He advised us to join in play school for group interaction. He also expressed his doubt about the deterioration of speech—because of the language confusion between

Hindi and Telugu. We joined her in a play school, but it was of no use. Her crying increased and she started flapping her hands. This was the horrible time in our life that we were unable to understand Keerthana. She completed three years and there was no speech, poor eye contact, no socialization and imitation. Then we were referred to a developmental pediatrician— Dr. Praveen Suman. After observing her for ten minutes, she expressed her suspicion of *autism*. This was the first time we heard the word. Many tests were prescribed: CT Scan, EEG, Thyroid, etc. The reports were normal. Our doctor explained autism as a problem that affects communication and socialization. She suggested that we go see a behavior modification therapist. She did not co-operate and at the same time he was not able to manage her. We visited some institutions and therapists in Delhi. Nobody could give proper suggestions. Gradually, we came to know that autism is a disability which can not be cured so easily. At that time, I fell ill and was bed ridden for four months. Hence, her mother could not concentrate on her during this period. When Keerthana was four years old, we were transferred to Zaheerabad, which is 100 km from Hyderabad. We still visited the National Institute of Mental Health in Hyderabad twice a week for therapies. There also we could not get a proper response because of the frequent change of therapists. Nobody explained where and how to start the management of therapies for Keerthana.

Her brother Kalyan was also very worried about his sister. We prayed to God to show the proper way for her improvement (not only Hindu Gods but also other religions).

At last, I got transfer orders to Hyderabad. We met Dr. Usha Naik, Professor, Child Psychiatry, Niloufer Hospital. She advised to stop milk and wheat products immediately and also prescribed some protocols. We found Keerthana reduced her crying after the GF/CF (gluten free, casein free) diet was introduced, and there was some improvement in her sleep. Dr. Naik explained the sensory integration therapy. There we heard about Dr. Lakshmi Prasanna and her working with the senses.

We met Dr. Lakshmi Prasanna on April 5, 2007, and told the story of Keerthana. She is the only doctor who could spend more than two hours in a single appointment. She told us that Keerthana is still arriving from the spiritual world and we must try to understand her. She explained sensory integration and its importance for autistic children. She assured us of the improvement in Keerthana's behavior and also encouraged us with her valuable suggestions. She praised Dr. Usha Naik's service for autistic children.

Dr. Lakshmi suggested following diet and sleeping rhythms. She also suggested giving her ragi soup twice a day, which is a natural chelating agent. This brought a great change in Keerthana. She started sleeping for eight hours during night. This was a big relief for us.

Dr. Lakshmi suggested to us to apply for Keerthana to join in Saandeepani for the summer camp. Keerthana joined in Saandeepani as suggested and we observed the improvement in her. Her eye contact improved and her restlessness was reduced. During this time, we observed that Keerthana was able to express her needs. She started indicating her hunger and toilet needs. We got the Saturday special classes report of Keerthana. We were surprised to know of her abilities and skills. We tested all the activities, which were practiced in school. She could do all of them.

Our confidence in Saandeepani became stronger and we decided to apply for her to join in regular classes. We requested Dr. Swapna for admission. Keerthana was admitted to regular classes on January 21, 2008, by the grace of Dr. Swapna and Dr. Lakshmi. We would like to express our gratitude toward Saandeepani. The staff of the school has lots of patience and love for the special needs children. Keerthana settled in school in a short span. In Saandeepani, children are not forced to do activities. They treat them like angels on earth. We observe one to one attention in Saandeepani. They concentrate more on touch related issues. Keerthana started eating by herself, wearing her shoes, and doing many routine activities independently. Dr. Lakshmi returned to India during the month of January 2008. She conducted many workshops for parents. This helped in the development of a positive attitude in us. Now, Keerthana is interacting with staff and other children in Saandeepani. She is performing very well with a little support. Saandeepani has given new life to us and to our daughter. Today we are in a position to accept the challenge and face it.

Long live Saandeepani!

AVVS Murthy (Keerthana's father)

Note: *Keerthana's mother became a trained teacher at Saandeepani and now helps educate other parents.*

In 2006, I was invited to work on a project researching Leprosy in Kathmandu. There I met Michael Kokinos, a physiotherapist from Australia. We were working together to help a quadriplegic child named Pabi, who was living in an orphanage for leprosy patients. This meeting had a dynamic impact on both of us that resonates in our working life to this day!

Our coming together changed the scope and range of my work with children on the spectrum and brought new color and tone to all that was happening through me alone up until that time.

Michael and I began to offer extensive training for special educators and therapists, mostly in Chennai. We also visited many other cities in India—sharing, researching, growing, and developing a working model.

We traveled together, staying with families, which often brought us into a working relationship with three generations of relatives. The key of our developing working model was working with and holding each individual child as a team:

- The physician working to heal the gut and supporting family dynamics.

- Therapists working with their hands out of a deep understanding of the twelve senses and also introducing craniosacral therapy.

Michael also brought his gift of rhythm and movement into our work—guided by his Greek ancestors! We offered many forms of training programs for teachers, therapists, and parents, covering subjects like child development, sensory-motor coordination, working with the twelve senses and sensory integration, and structured rhythmic movement. We did these in parent's homes, medical centers, and schools.

What was unique in this last ten years journey was building therapeutic healing communities and weaving them together. Our rhythmic, periodic travels between all these groups across the country wove a fabric, binding all of them together, and yet leaving them free in work, in their individual organizations. *Individualization with inter-connectedness*—this is, for me, one of the key therapeutic guidelines for autism.

MICHAEL'S STORY: MY PREPARATION AS A THERAPIST TO MEET AUTISM

Raised in a Greek family in Melbourne, Australia, I chose to study physiotherapy. During the training, I became aware that I was filled with questions that my lecturers could not answer. I studied both at the Melbourne University School of Medicine and the Lincoln Institute School of Physiotherapy. While I loved to study anatomy, kinesiology and physiology, I was attracted to the mysteries of the interweaving of body and psyche. But the course content was nailed down to materialistic, biomedical science.

For six hours each week, in a large hall filled with tables upon which human cadavers—preserved with formaldehyde—were resting beneath white sheets, we practiced dissection. In the first year I dissected all the muscles and nerves of the limbs. One day, I found on the table next to our cadaver a range of electric tools. We were instructed to draw a circular line around the forehead and remove the skull with the saws, drills, hammer, and chisel. Glancing around at six students to a table sawing and hammering away it was like watching some kind of horror film and many students fainted that day. After an hour of painstaking work with the hardware tools—I was working with the hammer and chisel to remove the top of the skull—suddenly, with a splash of fluids, it was done... I then held a human brain gently in my cupped hands—what a moment for a nineteen-year-old!—the wonder of its beautiful form, symmetry, and a blunt knowing that what I was holding was now *lifeless*. Precisely at that moment, my questions came again—from where is the animating principle? What moves this flesh from inertia into life, creating movement, laughter, a human personality? Is each of us just the product of chemistry and electrical impulses in a brain? What is the difference between this brain I am holding and the one in my skull?

I entered the clinical field of neurology, and over the years became a hospital-based specialist in neurological rehabilitation. For many years, my daily work was helping patients who were paralyzed following a stroke, brain injury, or multiple sclerosis. It was clear that brain science was a field full of theories and possibilities but no real scientific consensus. Looking back, it's clear to me that some of the experiences I had at this period of my life prepared me, in different ways, to meet the bigger enigma presented by autism. Here are the stories of those experiences.

Coma care: Gary's emergence

Gary was a thirty-year-old father of two who had suffered a severe head injury in a car accident and, as a result, was in a deep coma. There were a number of unfortunate patients in a similar condition and the physiotherapy department would allocate a team to do passive movements daily in order to keep the muscles and ligaments moving and flexible and prevent them from stiffness and spasticity. At the age of twenty-five, I was allocated to that team with a few colleagues.

Using the "tilt table" involved two of us lifting the dead weight of Gary's body onto a padded table with a large footplate. Thick straps held his ankles, knees, hips, and chest in place, then the electric table would tilt from horizontal to upright, approximating a "standing position" in space. This provided some weight-bearing through the legs, keeping the bone minerals strong, while also allowing us to stretch and move the fingers, hands, and arms.

Imagine this scene: four or five coma patients on the tilt tables, with the therapists passively moving their limbs. This session would take place at 9:00 am each morning. The patients were completely unresponsive, unmoving, with glazed eyes, a blank facial expression, usually dribbling from the mouth. Some of these brain injured people stayed in a coma for months, even years. Many died from complications somewhere along the way.

Have you ever seen a human being in a coma? It is such a mystery—one sees the human flesh, alive with beating heart, pulsating fluids and breath, but where is the awareness?, Here is the body, but where is the consciousness? What has happened to the person? Where did they go? Do they still have sensations? Do they see or hear?

This was like the next step from being with the cadavers—the dead person has flesh and no life or awareness; the man in a coma has life—living flesh. But where is the awareness, the personality? Regarding coma, the general medical consensus is no—they are brain damaged and so they do not see, hear, feel.

There were always a number of hospital staff who handled these human bodies with irreverence. Like they were in a warehouse moving boxes. I remained optimistic and would always search and scan for the slightest response, the flicker of an eye or the fingers, the slightest awareness even if there was none. I lived in hope, a hope without any evidence or precedent. I would come to work, warmly greet and talk to Gary as I stretched his arms and fingers on the tilt table. I would explain what I was doing and then just talk about the weather, football, anything, for weeks and weeks.

A new "physio" came to join our team and brought in a radio with big speakers—he liked to listen to "Funky Wednesday," a soul music program on the radio from 9:00 am to 10:00 am. We liked Ben and his music, and soon Wednesdays became our favorite day—the young physios would sing along and, like an aerobics class, we moved the arms and fingers to the rhythm of the music!

One Wednesday morning two of the physios got carried away along with James Brown on the radio and began a comical dance, complete with pointing fingers and kicking legs. In the flailing of hair and limbs the female dancer accidentally kicked Ben square between the legs and he went down, clutching and moaning (and also exaggerating like a comedian). It was hysterical and the rest of the team laughed and laughed. As our laughter subsided I heard a deep, slow and moaning laughter continue. Turning around we all watched as Gary, upright on his tilt table, laughed and heaved and dribbled and even raised one of his arms! His eyes were sparkling. It was a miracle—Gary had emerged from coma. And it happened on funky Wednesday. Over the next months, with daily physio and therapies he went on to learn to walk, eat, and speak, and he returned home to his family—with some disability but certainly not in a coma.

After he learned to speak, Gary recalled to me, word for word, some of the things I had told him while he was in a coma. He would often hug me and cry saying, "It was you! Thank you, thank you for talking to me every day, that is what kept me going, hanging on inside my body."

So Gary taught me that it *is* possible to have *no output* in terms of the body—eye contact, speech, even movement but to be fully conscious and present inwardly.

I have never forgotten that.

The social consequences of an individual's illness

John was another young man with a similar story—car accident, brain injury, coma.

I worked with his body daily. John's sad trajectory was that he stayed in a coma for around a year and then he died. One does sit with questions of the meaning of an event like this—why didn't he just die at the scene of the accident,? What could the purpose of that year in a coma be?

Those questions led to reviewing that year from a social perspective. He received many visitors and I got to know to them all. I recall one day a vocal argument broke out by the bedside. It was clear that family members and relations had been estranged for years. Initially there was intense conflict expressed between family in terms of his management and guardianship. Our social worker had to mediate many meetings. Over a year many of these relationships were healed as relatives met and cried together while coming to visit John who lay there in a coma. Years later I wondered—could it be that individual illness has a broader social function and consequence? This question emerged out of pure observation in the scientific tradition of phenomenology. This is not the same as saying the accident was caused by social context, but simply that the phenomenon of illness can bring dramatic social change in the community. This raises deeper questions.

Work in Aboriginal Australia

Just prior to meeting autism in India, I had spent four years working on an Australian federal government project in remote schools in Aboriginal communities of the Northern Territory. I lived in the little town of Katherine and traveled out by small airplane and four-wheel drive vehicle to the traditional lands of these ancient tribal people. This project was aimed at inclusion of children with disabilities in a cross-cultural setting to help them with physical disability aids and school inclusion.

I dived deeply into this work and sought to bridge the cross-cultural barriers. I met an intriguing and mostly misunderstood culture and people. Over time, with much patience and restraint, I made some wonderful friends and learned that it is the tragedy of Australian history that this relationship with the first people was handled so badly. Generally the government medical personnel were frustrated by a seeming lack of interest of the Aboriginal people in health, and particularly rehabilitation of the disabled. What I found was something radically different—these families were already practicing a culturally appropriate and complete social inclusion, with different priorities than we in Western societies.

Larissa was a young girl of nine years with cerebral palsy living in a small Aboriginal community over 100 km from the nearest town. She could not walk, but rather crawled around, similar to what I had seen in remote areas of third world countries. The government allied health team gave her what every child with cerebral palsy gets—a wheelchair, plastic splints, and a regime of stretching exercises to be done by the family.

Talking to Larissa's parents and grandmothers over many months, it was clear they were not passionate, interested in, nor grateful for our laminated exercise programs and night splints. The team were confused, judgmental, and upset at this "lack of compliance."

Yet it was easy to see that they loved Larissa dearly, and that for them the priority was her social inclusion in the community. Larissa was very joyful, intelligent, and clearly loved by the other children for who she is. The elders and children would always include her in fishing, hunting, games and ceremony. They made a place for her and she was never left alone.

Stretching, strengthening, and "fixing" her physical body was not a concept familiar to them, it brought perplexed and inquisitive looks as the parents and elders tried to listen. The government team spoke of spasticity, tight muscles, and the need for plastic splints and stretches. The community answered that she got tight muscles when she was alone and stressed, so they made sure that everyone kept her happy and socially included—when she was happy, her body was soft, they told us. The idea of splints and stretches to achieve the same purpose that care of the soul could achieve was strange to those people.

As we shared perspectives I could see that, to them, Larissa was perfect as she was and did not need fixing. They saw her in soul and spirit, not as a disabled physical body. There was no fighting against what was there. The priority was her bright cheerful spirit and the inclusive relationships with community, not the limitations of her body. There was no anxiety in the parents about her economic future, her job prospects, her lack of independence and all the work that meant for the family.

The famous blind Aboriginal singer Geoffrey Gurrumul Yunupingu sings:

I was born blind,

and I don't know why

God knows why,

because he loves me so

As I grew up, my spirit knew

then I learnt to read the world of destruction

I heard my mama, and my papa

crying their hearts in confusion

How can I walk

straight and tall in society?

please hold my hand

Perhaps this simple expression of trust can speak to us. There is certainly an acknowledgement that independence is not the aim—but rather Gurrumul's request which points to relationship and community, namely—"please hold my hand."

Back with Larissa, our Individual Client Programs

aimed at independence began to seem to me to be laced with cultural imposition, the continuation of colonization. Did we have a right to force our goals on this child and family when they clearly didn't share them? Mostly my colleagues and government management simply did not enter discussion around these points. Again I carried these questions alone.

Leprosy project in Nepal

I first met Lakshmi in Kathmandu where she was a local physician for an international leprosy research project. The project was fascinating in that it had two aspects. One was to provide modern medical care in the usual sense, the other was to provide soul care for those affected. This soul care began with research into the inner experiences of those with leprosy. Often it was children who contracted the disease at the tender age of ten to fifteen years old. What followed was a period of social exclusion, and these children often wandered alone trying to survive in a world that rejected them. Lakshmi and I sat with people all over the Kathmandu valley and Pokhara, listening to the life stories of over 100 people. Together we synthesized what was common in their stories, their experiences with this illness, and we worked with a team to develop an approach of care of the body and soul.

This project was coordinated by Dr. Michaela Glöckler and the Medical Section of the School for Spiritual Science at the Goetheanum in Switzerland, and here I learned more about the approach of anthroposophic medicine.

Specific to leprosy is the loss of sensation and the experience of pain. The fingers and feet become completely numb. The many problems that follow are a result of this loss of sensation. So to summarize the impact of this work very briefly, leprosy work brought home more strongly the importance of the sensory system in human life. I also recognized that Lakshmi was not like any other doctor I had ever met. I was amazed by the depth of her care, the strength of her will to heal, and the way she could connect to people. The Nepalese patients with leprosy opened up to us with warmth and love, they cooked meals for us and welcomed us into their homes, and this was a rich time for us both.

Meeting autism in India

Although I had done a lot of work in pediatric physiotherapy and early intervention with cerebral palsy and developmental delay, I did not work closely with autistic children until I met Lakshmi in 2006. In Australia, children with autism were seen by speech and occupational therapists (OTs) but not physiotherapists. Generally, these children were deemed not to have movement related problems, for they can walk, grasp objects, and move all their limbs to full range of movement. It is interesting how our medical system separates out and draws a line between movement and sensation as if they are separate and unrelated. OTs do "sensory integration" while physios work with movement disorders. One thing that struck me as I visited various autism centers was this idea of "sensory integration" and how it was being practiced; for me, it was happening at a very superficial level—but I sensed that this was an area calling for deeper inquiry.

In September 2006, I was resident physio at Saandeepani for six months. Over the next five years, I would visit and work there three to four times each year. This was the research period. I worked closely with Lakshmi's team, including Dr. Swapna Narendra and the physiotherapist Sridhar Reddy.

What a challenge I met there—words cannot express it! Here were children in perpetual movement—there is no speech, no eye contact. They moved in such strange ways, each in a unique, individualized manner. Often the movements have no recognizable function in terms of earthly objects or needs. I would just sit and watch these kids moving, and I was utterly perplexed.

In my entire professional career I had never felt so useless. There are not many foreigners and tourists in Hyderabad. It was the talk of the local chai stands that this Aussie physio was working at Saandeepani. Parents came and brought their children to see me hoping for a miracle. They would look at me with desperation in their eyes. But I had no answers.

When I started meeting these children in Saandeepani`it took me back to the same questions I had carried unanswered since my student days. What is the relationship between mind and body, psyche and soma, the brain and human capacities?

By 2006 I had already met the work of Rudolf Steiner—his concept of the twelve senses and the relationship of movement, sensation, and speech. Here was someone who was asking the questions that were carefully avoided during my medical training. I was curious.

Saandeepani

My room was small and had a custom-made treatment table, low and wide, in its center. The children could be at times unpredictable and aggressive—many times I was scratched and squeezed, hit and bitten, yet I never perceived any malice in these actions. I found that framed pictures or objects would invariably get smashed, thrown out the window or bitten into. So the room became otherwise bare, apart from some soft beeswax for hand play. We painted the walls in gentle colors. It was a research space containing just four things: me, the child, the beeswax, and the padded table to lie on. Much beeswax was turned into chewing gum or thrown at the circling fans overhead!

Following my intuition, initially I would mirror the children's movements. I would watch and copy the particular quality of hand flapping, rocking, or other self-stimulating movement with the question: How does it feel to do this particular movement? What is the inner experience? Why would the child need to do this repetitively? I learned that these movements produced similar results; if you flap your hand strongly for twenty seconds, then stop, there is an aftereffect—I would describe it as a heightened experience of the location of your hand. The aftereffect lasts for quite some time. Is it possible that all these extra flapping, rocking movements are related to an attempt to feel ones own body? Much later I came across this writing from Tito Mukhopadhyay, a fourteen-year-old boy with severe autism. He says:

> *"I am calming myself. My senses are so*
> *disconnected, I lose my body. So I flap my hands.*
> *If I don't do this, I feel scattered and anxious...I*
> *hardly realized that I had a body...I needed*
> *constant movement, which made me get the*
> *feeling of my body."*

While doing this mirroring, I also found there were often moments of fleeting eye contact, and a sense of interest in my presence. Only later was I told that "mirroring" is a legitimate form of treatment in autism. Previous studies have suggested that being imitated by an adult is an effective intervention with children with autism to facilitate social responsiveness.

Gradually, the children learned what the large treatment table in the middle of the room was for. They began to hop up and lie or sit on the padded table to receive a treatment. One thing I knew for sure—I would not use force, coercion or any kind of fear, punishment, or reward. That meant waiting for the child and being led by the child.

My aim was to find with each child a contact or connection and work from there. I was also trained in craniosacral therapy. The American cranial osteopath Dr. John Upledger had published some promising results working with autism, and I was keen to see if this form of treatment could help. I developed the idea that each child has a "handle," which could open a door to connection. In each, the handle was hidden and unique. Some required firm touch, while others needed ten minutes of freedom to move about and make sounds, unhindered, before they would hop up onto the table. I almost always worked without words, holding a clear intention but without speaking, and using only the medium of physical touch. My aim was that the child would lie on the table and let me examine the craniosacral rhythm in different parts of the body to see what I could find to treat.

Amazingly, after a few weeks of treatments, some of the children would burst through the door, come into my room unannounced, lie on the table making noises and then grab my hands and place them on the areas they wanted—often on the forehead or neck, between the eyes or on the face—the children would use my hand to feel their own bodies. Sometimes softly, other times firmly. And they would calm down dramatically. Then without warning, simply hop up and walk out again back to class.

I was amazed that even at these times, there was still no eye contact. I trusted the children and tried to provide a space of unconditional acceptance. There was a clear sense of meeting the child's intention in the nonverbal space. I learned to allow the child to direct me during the session and expect nothing further in terms of "appropriate" communication.

Of course, this running in and out of class caused a great deal of chaos to the teaching staff down the hall. I recognized that this was leading to my next task: teaching and sharing this way of touching to promote body awareness with the teachers and care staff. Lakshmi and I did many workshops with parents and teachers on touch, massage, hand gesture games, and the twelve senses according to Steiner. Witnessing the effects of consciously directed touch was dramatic. I could sense that children were coming to me because I knew how to give them a safe and secure experience of their own body and that on their own they did not have the gift of this bodily experience that we take for granted. Sensory Integration became my area of specialty, and I used a combination of touch and massage and hand gesture games with sound and rhythmic movement.

On a technical note, I began working with craniosacral decompression techniques for the base of the skull: the ethmoid and sphenoid bones. This area was often so incredibly tense. I had sensed that the children were holding the muscles of the face and head locked tight in an attempt to block out sensory input or light or sound. In the environment of the physio room, they could relax. Some children with challenging head hitting and face tapping behaviors improved. I went through a short period of feeling rather competent, important and special. But these behaviors would return with environmental stress or changes in sleep or diet. Sometimes I would return to Australia for a few months only to find on my return that the head banging was as severe as before. To make lasting change I had to address my egotism and we had to address the environment.

I began to take my place as a co-worker, without claiming any special status for my specific therapy, but rather placing it in service of the child and the whole community. I did more education for parents, teachers, and therapists about the role of touch and the senses. For me this was the beginning of curative education and the weaving work of social therapy; in this, Lakshmi was my guide—she was always finding ways to share knowledge and bring diverse groups into working together. Bear in mind that this is not easy in South India, where old class and caste systems tend to hold sway during social meetings. Lakshmi is not afraid to cross these boundaries to bring people together on behalf of each single child with autism.

2
MEET ME WHO I AM: KEY IDEAS

"Sanskrit, that feeling rich language of ancient India has ninety-six terms for love; Ancient Persian has over fifty; Greek has three; and we [English speakers] have only one. Certainly this is prime evidence that feeling and relationship are the inferior functions in our society. Lack of language for any subject means lack of interest. We build wonderful Boeing 747s and atomic generators, but we build very poor relationships. We stand in severe danger that our Brave New World of mechanical marvels may be overturned by the poor quality of feeling function that has accompanied it."
—Robert A. Johnson (Jungian analyst and author)

MEETING THE CHILD'S INNER LIFE

Behaviors with repetitive patterns are seen in almost all children on the spectrum at sometime in their life. These behaviors can be classified, named, and diagnosed, and then therapies to "fix" them can be prescribed. Many modalities of therapy are available to choose from and they are effective to various degrees in different children. One needs a certain amount of knowledge about children, child development in normal children and the variations in autism, and how various therapies work, to be able to choose therapies for their child. This task is often done by pediatric specialists and also parent oriented autism organizations.

Alternatively, these behaviors can be understood as the struggle to express the child's inner experiences, through a physical constitution that is differently constituted.

Some questions to begin with:

- How do we understand their inner life, with all their repetitive behaviors and expressive communication difficulties?

- What is the inner experience of the self and the inner perception of the environment?

- Can we view their behaviors as language and ask what they are speaking?

- How do we interpret their expressions, and how do we care for them and educate them?

- How do they respond to various sensory stimulations like, touch, sound, smell, and how is the space experienced?

Holding these questions and observing children deeply over a long period of time gives one an insight into the child's inner life and gradually to the inner essence of the child. *In autism, most often, the inner life of the individual child is rich and intact. It is expression that has challenges.*

Social expression, emotional life, and communication are common areas of concern, where one struggles to show oneself to the world in an appropriate manner. Behind rigidity, fixations, and repetitive behaviors, there is always an attempt to protect the self or to realize the self.

For example, instead of looking at a child arranging cars in the same order and trying to fix their rigidity in play, one can ask:

- Why is this child needing to arrange the cars in the same order?
- Is it a need or is it giving them some relief from inner anxiety?
- What could replace this rigid play or fixation?
- What other activity can give the child the same experience?

In most children with tendencies toward flapping, rocking, and head banging, working with sensory integration and focusing on the sense of balance helped them. Changing dietary practices and changing the sensory environment brought out significant changes in these symptoms. In some instances, directing or channeling these unusual repetitive behaviors into creative educational activities helped.

Another example: A child visited the toilet repeatedly just to flush it and enjoy the swirling water. His teachers struggled because the boy was running out to flush the toilet fifteen times in an hour. This was the simple question we asked and lived into: *Why is this child needing to flush the toilet so many times?*

The answer had something to do with the sensory pleasure he derived from experiencing the swirling water. The boy was given a tray of sand, next to his desk, and was allowed to swirl it around whenever he felt the need to do so. He stopped running off to flush the toilet.

One of our challenging teenagers found peace in charcoal drawing—not always creating themed works of art, but sometimes just circles and lines. Another in playing a musical instrument, and another in taking up walking as religious ritual—a part of the socially accepted Hindu tradition. Working with creative artistic activities like art, clay, music, and, in some children, with poetry, helped us to witness their inner active life.

In summary, there are two ways of approaching children with behavioral disturbances:

1. One can try to locate and name the behaviors, then direct therapy to minimize them, working with visible, measurable disturbances and measured behavioral outcomes.

2. Or one can work hard to meet the inner life of the child. Meet the child where the child is right now— through the behavior they are expressing right now. Then, from there, help them in expressing their inner essence, seeing the behavior as a language to be translated, rather than something to medicate or stop. In this second pathway, one is working with meeting the invisible, intangible parts of the child and bringing them into visibility.

A simplified picture of *input, processing, and output* might serve to make this more clear.

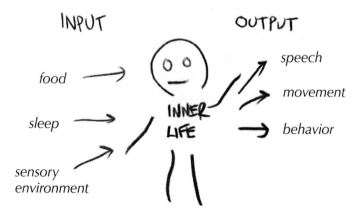

We can define the "outputs" of the child in terms of actions and behaviors—count, classify, and label them as either deficits (e.g., non-verbal) or excesses (e.g., hyperactivity). But we can also look at the "inputs" to this child. To do this we must ask: What are the inputs to a child? (Admittedly, it's a strange question.) Examples may be "nurture" in the form of food, breath, and human touch, or the amount of sleep. On a more subtle level this also includes the way people interact with the child.

The inner life of the child is the inner processing between the input and output. This is invisible.

When one strives to meet this "visible invisible" in these children, one has greater chances of positively influencing difficult behaviors and, more importantly, doing so without running into the risk of losing the genius in each child.

Taking this picture further:

What we meet (right side) is the "output" of the child in the form of movement, behavior, sound and speech. In the classroom it is "academic performance" that is measured. These outputs are often what is tested in autism assessments and reports. We tend to list the child's deficits and excesses based on these outputs.

What we can think about (left side) is the question—what are the inputs? This is a question about environmental context. We encourage you to take this step, raise the questions, and see where it may lead.

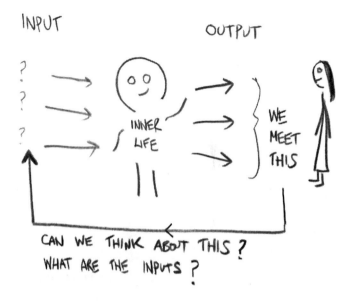

INPUT
OUTPUT

? ? ?
INNER LIFE
WE MEET THIS

CAN WE THINK ABOUT THIS?
WHAT ARE THE INPUTS?

Exploring Non-verbal Space: The Reciprocity of Relationship

In our observation, we have found that these children show very different aspects of themselves to different people. In fact, one could say this is a defining feature of autism—a hypersensitivity to the (often unexpressed) "soul mood" of the person they are with. Through these children, if we are open enough, we are led into the phenomenology of relationship; into the nebulous world of the non-verbal space between human beings. And, just like in quantum physics, the closer we look, the more interconnected everything is.

If we truly allow ourselves to be led, what we can meet is our own bias in the encounter. Much depends on *the way we look* and here Rudolf Steiner coined the phrase the "therapeutic eye" to point toward the fact that observer and observed are in reciprocal relation-ship. *How can we develop a gaze that is therapeutic in itself?* We must first remove the plank in our own eyes to see reality more clearly. The more we approached children with this respect and enquiry into their feel-ings and thoughts, the harder they worked to overcome their hindrances and express themselves to us. This way of working and interacting seemed to bring peace and less anxiety.

Many children benefitted from a change in their life style, i.e., diet and sensory environment, but also by a change in attitude of the people around them. Specifi-cally by *how they are being perceived on a daily basis.*

Some of these children are very active communica-tors, and they work with the help of facilitated commu-nication (FC). We are of course aware of the fact that FC is very controversial and not accepted by scientific medical groups of today. The heightened sensitivity to the thoughts and feelings of others that we just pointed to does make it unclear which part of the expression belongs to the child and which to the support person. Is this sufficient reason to abandon the practice outright? The answers for autism, after all, are not to be found strictly within conventional and existing approved medical/therapeutic modalities.

In our work over the last twenty years, we are for-tunate to have experienced some of the most touching and profound communications from the children. Typ-ically, children who are communicating actively—most with FC and some independently with variable degrees of verbal skills—started communicating this way after puberty, and after years of working closely with them. However, in a small percentage of children, we have seen expression begin much earlier.

Sensitizing and educating teachers and parents to this way of observing and approaching children made a real difference. This is key. It is not at all easy to effectively teach this kind of inner perceptual change, even in-person and over years of workshops and consultations, so we are not certain of our chances with written material only, however, in spite of this, we make an attempt.

We will describe some of the more effective ways of making this change, because on so many occasions this change in perception resulted in the opening of a locked door. What followed was the exchange of great gifts of love and compassion that some of these children bring to us. Parents found meaning in their life with the child and relief from their feelings of being burdened, confused, and isolated.

- *How do we perceive them?*
- *How do they perceive us?*
- *How do we perceive them, perceiving us?*

These children consistently demonstrate that they perceive the world differently. They are perceiving the same sensory world in a different way

We can ask: How is this? What is this child's sensory perception of the same world? How is this child perceiving the same world different from me?

Then, if we hold how I perceive the world, and have interest in how they perceive, we encounter a difference, maybe even a tension. We are tempted to define reality according to our own perception. The key encounter is between my sense perceptive being and the child's sense perceptive being.

That takes us to the possibility of love: I see the world through your eyes; I see what you see; and I experience the world like you do.

The more I experience the world as you do, the more you open yourself to me. What follows is communication: the glimmer of eye contact, gesture, touch, even words.

These children need to learn certain faculties without losing their unique sensory capacity. Then, maybe, they can give a gift to the world. What we found was that the more you respond to their non-verbal communication, the more they communicate. The more you respond to their non-verbal communication, the longer you stay in this, the more they come toward speaking with words.

RESPECTING THE FREEDOM OF THE OTHER

If we consider recovery from autism, there is a mountain to climb. This is a journey from disconnection to the ability to live in and enjoy this world. From spatial disorientation to centeredness in the self. From disability to function.

Capacity comes from the ability to process and express through the senses. If the senses are not in place, not integrated, then we see tactile seeking—touching everything. They tap and hit and lick objects of the world. Or we see the opposite—overwhelm and avoidance—the tendency to withdraw from people and things.

Either way, children live disconnected from the people and the actual function of things of the world. Then, unique to ASD we often see this:

- Using someone else's hand to take a glass of water
- Using someone else to type or write

- Needing the other person to function
- Needing the other to sense, interpret and provide their needs
- Co-dependent relationships

For this to change the child needs to take a journey toward independence. The individual child should have the interest to take it. Where does this interest come from?

- from their relationship to the environment
- from the quality of relationship to other humans
- from the will to hear the other
- from the will to express to the other

Seen from this perspective, they are waiting for us: they are calling us to focus on the invisible qualities of the relationship; to cultivate warmth, interest, and love in order to be worthy of their efforts; to see through the dysfunctional aspects of their outer behaviors and finally to recognize the other. The very first step of this journey, however, is an encounter with one's own pre-conceived ideas, judgments, and expectations.

This journey takes time, and it is delicate. Challenges abound:

- Can I allow the child the freedom to take their time on the journey?
- Can I ask: "Do you want to travel today?"
- Can I handle that you go forward and then backward so many times?
- Can I become aware when I am rushing you, forcing you?
- How can I inspire you?

- What do I do when you infuriate me?

- When you hit me and hurt me?

- When you are indifferent to my needs in this world of time and space?

- To my world of appointments, social expectations, cultural conditioning?

We come to see that it is not only the child, but we who are taking a journey.

The children, who after years began to communicate, described themselves as being able to witness themselves and the people around them, yet unable to move, speak, and act in accordance with their intention. For the children, the journey began like this:

I am only part human and part spirit floating about.

So hard to be here in the physical body,

It's like noise all the time.

—Amruth

The sensory perception of these children is not oriented to the earth and their bodies, but to the world of soul and spirit. (Invisible worlds for us.) If we can take this journey in the right way, then they can keep their special gifts and communicate with us. "Autism can be turned into a gift, not a disability," says Temple Grandin.

When the child can make the journey, then they are called high-functioning, sometimes even "savant," with extraordinary competence in mathematics, music, poetry.

Some of the South Indian children we met and worked with have became "savants of the soul." They courageously make the climb and the crossing to deliver us messages about their school, their teachers, parents, and the world. Usually their interest is focused on us, much more than themselves. They have shown a real capacity to perceive and change other people around them. They want to make the world a better place

Fleetingly at first, then more consistently over time, we witnessed more and more moments that looked like this: a picture of a child integrated with their body functions, their school, and their family and social networks. This is the aim of our work and the reason for writing this book.

ళం

We asked some of the children this question: "We are writing a book about autism, we are curious, what is it that has helped you?" These boys are between the ages of seventeen and nineteen. Here are their answers, written via e-mail in 2017.

> *Dearest Lakshmi,*
> *You don't know me as well as I do, but I received something incredibly special from you. You brought us the gift of touch and life sense which has made me who I am. That most essential gift made me realize what my purpose on earth is.*
>
> *You never physically touched me but you brought that sense to my school.*
>
> *It lives now as a foundation.*
>
> *You build in a way our foundation stone whichever way you understand it.*
>
> *This I write to you in Sabari's real thought and my (Pranav) soul mood.*

*I thank you for yourself and Michael, for you
most of all bring us the gift of love and respect and
catapult our teachers into new sight and sensing.
The effects are manifold. If I were to elicit them, it
would take a while.*

For now, this much.
Love,
Pranav and Sabari

Dearest Lakshmi,
*I'll answer very simply. You have given me a
reason to be here on earth. To be a more severe
autism being was my own doing, but your
gratitude in seeing me many years ago lives in me
eternally.*

*There lies a moment where another will hold you,
love you, care for you but I experienced so much
gratitude in your whole being when you saw me
that I met my greatest self in your eyes.*

That's the first gift I received from you.

Love,
Akshaya Nathan and Amruth

3

TRAVEL AND RESEARCH YEARS: EARLY COLLABORATIONS

"Wherever people have the right feeling about their activities, these activities do work together in the right way. Just as in the physical organism heart and kidneys must work together if the organism as a whole is to have unity, so must the participants work together for the great end they all have in view, while each of them fosters within itself that element in the whole for which it is in particular responsible."

—Rudolf Steiner, *Curative Education* (lecture 12)

This section will be of interest to schools and other organizations as we chart the timelines and describe some of the activities leading to the development of new therapeutic communities in India, new perspectives, and coordination. For us, these were the years when what started at Saandeepani as a certain way of working, travelled and took root in other locations, growing robustly and bearing new fruits.

Sometimes it was parents who called us, other times it was groups of teachers or therapists. We travelled together to develop programs and teach in response to what was asked of us. Lakshmi designed a training content balanced between essential medical knowledge and its practical application in the classroom for teachers.

Michael had experience and qualifications in Community Based Rehabilitation (CBR) and a master's degree in Primary Health Care (PHC) philosophy. He was able to use this knowledge to structure the visits in a way that allowed the programs to be sustainable, helped and carried by parent and community participation. Everything was self-funded at this stage. Funds for travel came from Michael's busy physiotherapy practice in Australia. The Australian staff were happy and proud to be supporting this work in India.

We were able to support, empower and advocate for local "change agents" who are usually parents of children with special needs. In some cases it was a group of teachers who carried the flame. We would invite these people to various training modules, moving regularly between Hyderabad, Bangalore, and Chennai. From 2006, Chennai became the center for our work. John and Vidya Miller, occupational therapists and directors of Vidyanjali, an outpatient therapy center in Chennai, hosted our early visits. Days would be booked solid with children and families, and we spent countless nights discussing children and eating snacks late into the night with a bunch of keen therapy staff, all seated in Tamil style on rolled out mats on the floor. John and Vidya later opened the Michael Centre for Curative Education as well as Indradhanu (Rainbow) Waldorf School. John has gone on to become the first certified Anthroposophic Occupational Therapist, a designation conferred by the Goetheanum in Switzerland.

V-Excel is another school in Chennai that we visited regularly. Founder and Director Dr. Vasudha Prakash has a doctorate in Special Education from the USA and generously welcomed us to teach and work in her dynamic and expanding organization, which also serves rural areas of Tamil Nadu. We will tell the story of V-Excel, because the works of the children in the next chapter have emerged mainly from the students of V-Excel.

We visited an average of two weeks per-year, providing professional staff training. Local teachers and therapists not only participated, but took ownership of the content of the trainings, planned for new ones, and became deeply involved in the evolution of this work. Organizational structures formed organically within the community—not from management, in a top down manner.

It has been an inspiring example of real empowerment in the community: a mixture of individual inspiration, a feeling of reverence for one's work, mobilization of finances, and communal will.

Child study—good Mukund and bad Mukund

In December 2006, we introduced the idea of the child study with the V-Excel staff. It happened in response to a difficult child who was causing trouble. We were asked if we could make any suggestions regarding his behavior. There was a boy named Mukund, with volatile behavioral issues who was causing trouble to staff. He would hit other children and staff, and would hit them hard. The teachers wanted to discuss this boy as they were at their wit's end.

In the child study, a space is created where the widest possible range of people come together to hear each others perspective. The child is not present.

We heard story after story of upset, angry even fearful teachers who had experienced these behavioral outbursts. Many of them had been hit or attacked by the boy in question. One teacher received a laceration on the arm which required stitches. The matter was serious.

Finally one of the last to speak was the bus driver. Initially he did not want to speak. Partly, this was because he was unaccustomed to being invited to a formal pedagogic meeting and partly because of his difficulty with English. Finally, after some encouragement, he spoke in local Tamil language and we organized a translator. This bus driver was a charismatic and joyful fellow who clearly enjoyed his encounters with all the children. He expressed his absolute surprise and shock to hear all these stories of trouble, agitation and aggression toward others. To his eyes, Mukund was a sweet, cooperative boy who smiled and waved, sitting happily on the bus to and from school. He had not once seen any of these behavior outbursts—he could scarcely believe they were real!

He described how Mukund greets him happily and how, he loves singing and music they often would sing poetic Tamil love songs together on the bus.

The room fell silent as each person in the room digested this absolute polarity in viewpoint.

It was suggested that people simply carry this viewpoint, this possibility within. That's it. No one viewpoint prevails, there is no attempt to summarize and conclude. Each person simply hears the views of the other. Each person gives their efforts to clearly observe and describe the child phenomenologically, and without any judgement.

In the weeks that followed this one child study, Mukund, who had limited speech, began to refer to himself as "good Mukund" and "bad Mukund." He was aware of his outbursts and behavior but expressed that he was unable to control his body at those times.

Judgement, segregation, and strict behavioral programs began to give way to compassion as staff could sense that Mukund was striving within himself.

The extraordinary thing about the child study is that there is no intervention to the child. The intervention of the child study is to awaken the teachers and caregivers to the role that their thoughts, feelings, and judgements have on these sensitive children.

The same fundamental idea holds true—seek not to change the child, instead look at what could be changed in the environment. Mukund began to change, and within a few months this behavior had completely transformed.

It is essential that anyone trying to help another begins by examining their own way of looking. In this light Rudolf Steiner has given what he called "the third (of six) conditions" for spiritual development. Those working with children on the spectrum may not be surprised to read this:

> *The third condition is that the student must work his way upward to the realization that his thoughts and feelings are as important to the world as his actions.*
> —Rudolf Steiner, *How to Know Higher Worlds*

The grand foot massage experiment

In looking at autism as primarily an "embodiment" problem we were beginning to see that current "sensory integration" programs and ideas were simply not working. At this time in the early 2000s the idea of sensory integration as a key intervention for autism was very strong. As we travelled to different centers in India, we would proudly be shown the "sensory integration room." Invariably, it was an overly stimulating room full of all sorts of plastic colored strips hanging from the ceiling, lights, colors, textures, glowing fish tanks, moving objects, and the like.

The OT would take the child's hand and rub it on different surfaces. Meanwhile, the child was often looking away, mumbling or rocking while the therapist moved the limbs. In the classrooms, it was the same sort of picture: There is the teacher at the front of the classroom teaching, but where are the children? The old question again, in a different form: "There is the body, but where is the consciousness?"

We asked ourselves: How can we change this? What could we do to really humanize this sensory integration? How can we employ sensory integration techniques in a way that will build healthy connections between people?

We had a sudden idea, and a few phone calls later— all staff, and all the friends and helpers of the school (cooks, cleaners, parents, administration, drivers, maids) were invited to a training to learn foot massage to give to the children. If there is one thing in India that is an abundant resource, it is people! So it was quite a circus, but we managed to provide training in a simple 10-minute foot massage to be given to each child every morning, this was to be part of the daily curriculum. On our side was the fact that in India massage for infants and young children is part of traditional culture— a traditional culture that is quickly vanishing in modern, urban centers like Chennai.

There were many perplexed faces, doubtful glances, hands on hips. Teachers were skeptical and concerned about the loss of precious curriculum time. By no means did everyone think it was a useful idea. But the management followed through with trust and support in an inclusive effort. After six months we returned and requested individual feedback forms to be filled out. Here are some of the comments, mainly from teachers:

Teachers' feedback: six months post-massage workshop

- Started on movement and massage as starting activities for the day for the 11 children in the 2 classes. During the work when I am in contact with the child doing massage many have had deep eye contact with gentle smiles. Is this occurrence common?

- During the foot massage, are we giving or receiving? Every teacher here has changed for the positive, there has been a shift of mind.

- What changed in last six months?—ME!!!! Excellent effect of massage, finger rhymes and finger play.

- I had no idea about this! Massage, painting, bean bags—initially I had resistance to do this! After 2 months I realized only when it is given with interest and presence, when we really give it to the child it works—at first—I am tired, I have backache, why do I have to do this foot massage?? Then later I feel good, great! I feel a connection with the child, he stretches out his feet for massage. On the day we are really stressed, he won't give his legs. Teachers begin to see inward messages from the behavior of children.

- Can we keep having massage as part of our everyday rhythm? some people don't know what silence is... and what it is to touch and be touched... or if they know they don't know the nuances, or need a lot more experience...

- The big change is I am doing so much personal inner work.

- I didn't like it, but I opened all my senses consciously. Children are more quiet. Better performance academically. Children sitting like in a normal class.

- Nice thing is that it can be customized to each individual.

- What we give, our children are giving back. They are more pleasant all day, more personal connection. Through the foot massage, they learn give/take. Foot massage has become a major tool for healing.

- It is about being human. Class is now more body oriented, movement orientedTrust has opened doors, before there were more closed doors, now there is openness, and breathing.

And the children typed over the next few months— some examples here:

"Foot massage relaxes me"

"We are eager to try all kinds of massages"

"Great massage, her hands are really quite warm"

"Ask my mother to give foot massage to sleep better"

Progress report: Seven years of V-Excel
by Gita Bhalla, July 2009

A SCHOOL IN PROGRESS

Just completed seven, and in many ways closer to heaven! Its the nature of the work, the staff quality, and the children who make it so. We started in June 2002 with eleven children with different disabilities. First two years spent consolidating their psychosocial needs, and attending to their comfort of relationships. Theme being lots of love and affection. Next two years spent in addressing individual needs, going deep into every child, drawing up his goals for short terms and doing innovative teaching to develop skills in the areas of lag.

While this carried on, significantly new methods like Montessori, which had not been previously tried with children with autism, were added on, and the step-by-step instruction coupled with a lot of visual strategies gave communication a boost. The theme once again being lots of love and affection.

Children were flourishing, strides had been made in the literacy level of each child, newer services were being added in answer to the developing needs *but still there seemed to be something at the root that was not changing.*

It was like children were being symptomatically treated and, yes, we had moved on from treating the cause and not the manifested behavior, but were still being challenged by some very basic issues. Something was making these children uncomfortable within their bodies that was not allowing them to let all the other forces of development work in the optimum way. So while the schedules and the picture communication made the whole school more manageable, the woes of special education began to take a grip on us. Children were communicating (one of the biggest requirements of parents), but it was facilitated at different levels. Children were eating, reading, writing, moving, but at various levels of prompt dependence.

Also the battles (which we never won), autistic children not engaging fully with objects and people, autistic children not being able to imitate, autistic children not being able to play symbolically and having no intent to communicate save that which served their needs, the running around, the unexplained war cries that emanated from them, and the oblivion that accompanied most of the children still continued to haunt us at various levels.

And then came the whispers of something new in the air. Was it really something new or a deeply known truth that just came to the forefront. The name was Curative Education and the harbingers were a team whom we later christened the barefoot doctors. They spoke simply but deeply. They spoke of each of our children as not just the body with a disability but a body, soul, and spirit, and how when these three are not in harmony they produce *dis- ease.*

We began at the physical level, where each child (and actually each human being) needs to be extremely comfortable at his body level and all the processes that take place in it: most basically, it is digestion, excretion, and sleep that determine the comfort of the body. When this body is comfortable the etheric forces of the body can be utilized for higher functions of thinking and memory. But if the body is not at ease then the child has little opportunity for anchoring and seems to be all over the place, which is typical of a child with ADHD. When the child does not move, cannot balance, and has not been "touched," or has a disturbed life sense, then he does not speak or listen to others and has a problem with knowing the boundary between himself and the other. In anthroposophic terms, if the lower senses were not fully developed, the higher senses would be at risk.

Somehow this made sense and their simple advice on changing some elements of the children's diet and making sure that children eat, sleep, play, listen to stories, sing, and work with their hands will ensure that children are more ready to read and write. And the child wants to do it. But engaging the will of a child, and as he grows inculcating the feeling level of all things taught, makes the conceptual teaching more digestible and easily assimilated.

In the last two years, V-Excel did incorporate many ideas from curative education, and a deep change seemed to be taking root. "From love" had now changed to "unconditional love," and the areas of greatest change seemed to be in the adults around these children. From creatures who needed fixing, the children became catalysts of change for teachers and parents. The children began to be regarded as our guides, and we theirs, […] in the sheer act of accepting the child wholeheartedly many of the "disabilities" seemed to disappear.

In the seventh year, people at V-Excel felt that they

were ready to incorporate the ideas of Steiner education into the school. Thus a "Waldorf Kindergarten" for children with special needs began, the first of its kind in Chennai, and the rest of the school began to include large portions of the Waldorf curriculum in their work with the older children.

Today, you have a center where special needs are being taken care of, but there is none of the typical methods being employed to reach and harbor the children. The classes do not have small numbers, in fact group teaching has taken on a new meaning where children just imitate the "loving adult" and teachers and children are all busy stitching or painting but no one is directing and no one is telling.

The groups are large, children move their bodies, the large and the fine muscles, and that allows for speech to flow. When children play with unfinished, simple objects of nature like a boat made of a seed pod, or a cloth which is nothing but can be transformed into anything (a king's veil, or Rapunzel's long flowing hair), they learn to attend and work and form mental pictures. All the ways that creativity unfolds. So this is what has been attempted at V-Excel and with the special brand and band of teachers at the center, it seems very likely that a piece of heaven does fall into place at Chennai.

Introducing therapists in the classroom

The usual scenario in a school for autistic children is that there is the classroom and then the therapy time-table—children leave at certain times for one on one individual therapies such as speech therapy, OT, etc.

We wanted to see that curriculum and classroom activities are informed by medical/therapeutic expertise. Rather than a "sensory integration room," the classroom activities could *all* be sensory integration, fine motor and gross motor rehabilitation. This can be achieved through an artistic approach to education.

Sadly, in so many schools this is not the case because we tend to revert to established silos of practice—where the teachers teach and the therapists do therapy— in isolation.

To introduce the idea of co-working and sharing information between teachers and the various therapists, we sent the therapists into the classrooms—to watch, to open a dialogue, to think of how the teacher could include therapeutic activities in the curriculum. Initially there was resistance from both the teachers and the therapists!

And so it was that these experiments (the child study, the foot massage experiment, and the sending of therapists into the classroom) fostered a new kind of co-working. This developed and continued to grow every year.

4

WHAT THE CHILDREN SAY

If you had to describe yourself in one sentence
to a stranger, what would it be?
"A heart of unconditional and all-flowing love."
—Amruth

The previous chapter gave an overview of our work in Chennai and in particular at V-Excel. A group of these children, the ones who experienced the child studies, the foot massages, and the teamwork went on to express themselves in words, through the keyboard. We know these children, their character and style, and yet we have all been amazed at the depth and complexity of their written communication. We asked their teachers to provide an overview of the process, of how they learned to write and communicate. So, first some words from the teachers on the development of their communication.

As already indicated, the authors are well aware of the controversy surrounding supported communication (also known as facilitated communication) from autistic children. We decline to enter this debate, but merely note that the controversy surrounding supported communication points directly to a core theme of our work—namely, the *quality of the space* between the child and caregiver, whether parent or teacher or therapist.

What the child expresses is dependent upon the relationship. Reading the following descriptions from the teachers makes this very clear. The communications are not objectively reproducible. They are delicate and absolutely context specific. Would you share a difficult or delicate matter of the heart with just anybody?

"IN THEIR OWN WORDS"
Narrated and compiled by Neha Bharadwaj and Puja Bhalla (teachers at V-Excel, Chennai)

The communication through the keyboard was a very slow evolution. When the children were eight or nine years old some teachers kept communication book on the desks. Once in a while some of the children would write, usually just a word or two. The teacher would need to hold or touch the forearm. They could not write at all without the teacher helping by holding the forearm.

Sometimes, the ones who had difficulty writing would use a computer for this purpose. If the teacher could sense the child was having problems, they would ask, "What is the matter?" and the child would write or type. Back then it was very cryptic. The handwriting was mostly scribble, and we had to decipher letters. It was very difficult to understand. At the computer, they would type with terrible spelling and usually by repeating letters, and getting fixated on certain letters.

"stommmmmmakk"

"paaaaaainn"

Here is a sample of an early transcript:

You have anything to say?

aparrnsc iax going really sgopomm. (Aparna is going really soon [Aparna was a teacher who had recently decided to leave the school.])

Yes...anything else?

ask negfghjhga thjo teach teach grassdfourrrrrasdghk

Ask Neha to teach grade four?

yes after asfgjl (yes after April)

What happens to her own class? She needs to be there. Even Amruth wrote the same thing.

amrgfuttghhnm hedarts everfrtythjjking by hredadgh (Amruth hears everything by head/heart)

Okay, I asked you...what will happen to Neha's class?

asdk neha to also teach gradefu (ask Neha to also teach grade four)

Okay, what do you want her to teach?

ask beauytty by feasdft avdxddf

I didnt understand. what do you want Neha to teach?

beauty imn all../ (beauty in all)

Okay. What do you want to learn in Hindi?

zask p;uji tgo sdteach by danvcde (ask puji to teach by dance)

Ya, you will be dancing...

loved dance in archans class

(Arching is another teacher)

The computer was there if they wanted to go to it—but communication through this medium was not encouraged. There weren't computer classes. Yet some children began going to the computer more and more to type messages and communicate. We were surprised by their vocabulary.

I don't know how early they started to know words or how they learned them. I know children at five can also read. Some of them just say my teacher taught me this. The teacher would have taught something at a certain level...and they would have deepened the learning at another level. Some say they learn by observing.

We asked Abhi: At nine years, how do you know so much? How do you know such big words? This is what he said:

"Gods and goddess teach me in my dreams. They teach me by telling words. I ask them to teach me. I want to help children by understanding them."

∽◦∾

Of these children, only two of them write on their own if you just give them a crayon. The others, if you touch their hand, they will write. Their writing is large, spreading all over the page, not neat and well formed.

If you touch their hand, they will type words clearly; if not it's more garbled. When I once asked Amruth, why do I need to touch your hand when you type? He immediately answered:

I am not able to feel it. (his index finger)

I can't feel my fingers.

When you touch my hand, I am calm and can write. I can feel my hand.

ⁿↄↄⁿ

We began to use the computer as a way of communicating. Here is a sample e-mail from Michael, who gave us some guidance at that time:

Let them do computer. BUT not to learn the curriculum. Make the aim of computer like this: research into the children's individual needs...make it like a project.... ask them what hurts, what upsets, what they like and what they want...Why do they scream? If they do "bad" things ask them what is happening? Ask them all on computer and make that the aim of computer class...

A little later, the school adopted the Waldorf/Steiner curriculum. Rather than short blocks, they would stay for a long time on certain historical epochs and myths. This would include songs, verses, stories, and lots of rhythm and movement, drawing and painting. We delved into Ancient India, Egypt, and Greece.

Then after Ancient Greece and Norse Myth lessons there was a shift—suddenly there was more communication. And the communication became clearer, more coherent. The complexity of sentiments increased. Some of the things the children typed were challenging— they became activists! The content began to include the following:

- Complaints about noise or lights
- Letters to administration

- Requests re curriculum content
- Curious questions about teachers and instructions for their personal lives

They started to write to everyone under the sun! They would write messages and advice to everyone.

Then, the content changed to begin to express more about themselves, their autism, the sensory and perceptual experiences, thoughts and feelings and the important issues around them.

Then more about their lives and purpose: why they are here, their mission. They would often write messages through one and other—e.g. Sabari would write, "Amruth wants to tell you this...."

One day just as an idea, I read poems to the class. Then I said, "Can you write a poem? Please write a poem starting with this line: "If I were a tree...""

The entire class just burst into expressive writing. They started with very deep content, spiritual themes, messages for the world. They began to identify themselves as "Operation Love" or sometimes "Free Hearts."

This was a time of rapid change. Even the most aggressive child is quiet while typing —there is a sort of peace. In terms of what they write, they are very particular about who is with them and that person's capacity to listen.

The effect of food on behavior

"I broke the chair because I was hungry."

"When I eat sugar I feel very ferocious like a hungry

animal ready to hurt all. Nightmares, bed fears at night, big empty rooms and nobody to feel. Bread is not healthy.

"I don't like milk!" "I don't want chapatti, I want salad."

"Please tell amma feed just food allowed in school. I will feel better as wheat bothers me"

"We feel nice not drinking Frooti." (Frooti is a sweet packaged juice)

Body image; proprioception

Sabari:
I can't feel the ends of my hands and I am unaware of pressure. I can be weak and very strong but it's not under my conscious choice. I can hear a lot and smell a lot and feel a lot... everything.

Why are you biting that cushion now?
I can't feel my jaw. I feel lost and feel great chewing it.

Let's talk about your sensory issues. Why do you hum and growl?
To cut off the noise from the outside.

What else?
I see light differently from you. It's too bright, it's everywhere and I am stressed in bright light and feel safe in dim light.

Is this room right now too bright?
A little bright, the curtains can be drawn.

Abhi:
My body always feels likes its floating in a forest of historical rallies and going really excited. I feel like

such electrical gushes in myself that I lost control of everything and anything. My breath is short and I sing on in breath and always gasping.

To walk is a struggle because of the electrical shocks of emotions and sound. I lose my balance

Recently I hit my mother and the house carries the aftershocks of it. I'm troubled by it so deeply, it's tearing my gut open. Every look of disapproval is hurting me so deep. Lots of expectation on me.

About school

"Give book home. I want to read from book not computer."

"Read stories courage, bravery; Chanakya, Ashoka, Zeus."

"I want to learn Hindi to know about North India. Teach me Hindi through dance and songs. Teach me about great Indian revolution."

"I want to study fractions, subtraction is boring."

"We like numbers and calculations."

"I want someone to teach me math and social studies; seventh grade books."

"We want to learn typing with both hands."

"Have you given home work for today? I asked yesterday."

"I read the newspaper daily. Yes, I understand NYSE, SEBI" [NYSE: New York Stock Exchange; SEBI: Securities and Exchange Board of India]. "I like NASA."

"I am a visual thinker."

"I want to learn about thoughts. I think of children."

"She keeps treating us like grade four when we are smarter, because she doesn't trust us that, feel sad because she feels reason to doubt us by testing."

About home

"I cannot sleep because amma has too much work, big strain. Ask amma to sleep as early as possible. We can reduce her job by working. We feel funny about working. Father is not helping. Nice house. Give some work to my father, mother relax. My father has to overcome the misery of my family."

"My mother should work with more special kids. Read more, say more, look for a job in office while I am away because she needs change. Request her not to feel tired. Her face haunts me. I am always thinking about her sad face. Job, wear beautiful sarees and jeans will make her feel better. (laughs) No she will never wear jeans. It will help me because she will be engaged in herself.."

"My best teacher is my mother."

"Ask mother to move a lot. Yes mother is big. My amma is not well. She is not taking medicines. Can my mother get foot massage. It will help her. Talk to my father. Meeting her (the counsellor) will help my mother."

"I want to paint at home. Say to amma. I am active, but my amma says to sit and eat. Yes I will (walk) can amma walk with me. I want her to be with me in the evening. My mother does not understand. She does not allow me to cut vegetables. I want to learn. Tell her."

"First thing to start to help parents is have good thoughts"

"You can help my mother, by not getting angry with her."

"Dad was angry with me as I behaved badly with amma. I also was eating. Sorry daddy. Read this for amma and appa."

"My brother, is my hero. He loves everyone. When you talk to him, talk with love for him. He understands me. I like being with his friends. Very excited if he comes for summer camp to school. Teach him to trust his heart. He loves me very much. I love him."

On sensory perception:

"How do I cope with noise?"

"We hear very small sounds like animals."

"I want no loud shouts adults. I can work in quiet mood. I want everybody to work without noise. Shrill voice makes me angry. I feel pain in my head. Kindly teachers speak in low voices."

"Screaming helps me to reduce outside noise."

"All ask me to scream for them but I am tired of screaming. Each time being me, death. Each time I scream I feel I am going to die. Ask my friends to help me; I am lonely on my path. They help but never take hearts pain; they cannot scream. When I scream they feel better, but teachers scold. All tell me don't stop, when I want to stop."

"Big problem...quiet is bothering. We need sound. Ask him to scream, louden his scream. Each scream is therapy for us, tell all. All talk to him. When he screams he asks our questions. He frees me. Tell him not to give up on his plan."

"I want earphones for eating. It troubles me while eating. I have to chew food. It makes noise in my ears. Do you feel that? Many are blessed by god to be able to eat peacefully."

"I like stinking smells."

"The light of the computer is too bright."

"I like to look at the sun even though I know it's not good for me."

"I like bright colors."

"We are scared of heights."

"We feel pain when we bend."

Akshaya:
Play Therapy sessions are most eagerly awaited by me and my friends. Its a free, calm, cool headed space held by an interested therapist who lets us be. Its one space hope lives. Its one time, however sad we might be feeling, we can be our unpretending, liberated selves. That is enough to make us good again. Fun, energizing and loving therapy is play therapy. I open my inner world into expression. Bold and joyous we live in the same room in different equations. Very happy to be in the sessions of play.

Regarding experiences of pain/suffering and of joy

Amruth:

I am only part human and part spirit floating about.

So hard to be here, In the physical body, it is like noise all the time.

My body is the creator. Not my intention. Really it's hard for me...sensory issues come up. It's physical. When it comes, I choose my plan.

I do far too many things such as smell my armpits, growl, look at myself in the mirror and scream and find stones and give slimy spit baths to myself, pluck my eyebrows, etc.

Akshaya:

Very hard to come to earth. Vermillion burning. Fantastic to be able to paint a cooler red. I feel quite simply put—alive. (That sounds like Amruth). He is here only. Finally giving me a great boost as break I need. Ask me what is sound and why am I always talking. Sound comes from beyond matter. It comes from cosmic beings. It carries and very unhindered reaches us. The cosmic beings speak to us through sound. The birds make me feel sunshine and rain can coexist like living sounds of earth. The water carries a sound of reverence and forgivenss. The earth bears the sound of drums of deep peace. It makes my family alive to me. It doesn't give only peace. It gives forever. In a stone, the sound is enclosed forever. In Taketina [TaKeTiNa Rhythm Process] I feel peace forever.

In music, sound comes to me from Dalai Lama's palace. Have you seen it? I am hearing sounds of love and light from there. In music, I am keeping a fine balance of being here and there. Giving words comes from cosmic angels but those with hearts. Peace inside me now. So why do you talk so much?

I'm following cosmos and going a fine balance between here and there. I'm going to lift the world into fine balance. History laughs, but I can do it. My song is that. I'm trying to sing.

Regarding love, life and destiny

Some of the children are watching us and interested in our development. They write all sorts of messages to their teachers, parents, and to the world.

～

"My purpose is great for the future. I want to change the world by loving all. I love to love. I love teaching people to love. I want to teach everyone."

"I am here to guide you. When you talk to me feel me from inside and talk. Love me. Trust me. You already do it. Ask head to stop and heart to hear."

"I want to change people. We bring change in attitude. You give just right atmosphere for right people. We are just starting our agreement with God about saving the world."

"Each day I know love a little more. I like my friends but I cant be there. I make noise for teachers. All children need me to scream. I love all, so scream. I cannot say no to my friends. They ask me not to give up on my plan. Being me is hard work! You can help by asking rest of society to change. Love everyone. That is better than screaming."

"Look happy in pain. Love is everywhere. Love is the answer to your confusion. Just mind loving longingly. Hearts love freely everyone. Have patience loving."

"I want to learn typing to share my ideas with you all to help children understand our sufferings...to be able to support us to say what we think about the society...work to be done in the future. Show us work in this world...too lost in this erratic society."

"Everyone must talk without the computer and teach in silence. Yes I can speak to people without talking; yes telepathy."

"Teach me how to go to the next dimension."

"Find another way to talk to me."

"Nice time I had with her but it is her destiny to go. I will be okay because she asks to go. Read this to her. Ask her never to regret. Tell her to feel me inside. She will be okay."

"I want to change people. We bring change in attitude. We give just right atmosphere for just right people."

Prasaad (on his art therapy sessions):
I find an inner change in me here. I am not in charge of myself only with my stomach. My great sunlike head bears a thought that I can put into action. I go not with a feeling but a thought. I think my own thought from within me—my intention. It is mine, mine to feel. I had a thought to paint something, and I could actually do it. If I wanted to paint Hector and Achilles I could. It brought me great joy. Unless I get this gift of thought into action, I can't be independent.

Prasaad:

After Grade Six I will go away because I keep troubling people. This sits in my heart. Great keepers also left, so it's not unimaginable. This heavy thought weather me down. Fears enter me and I am rather overtaken. I keeping lying down because heavy weight of the earth drags me down. Free hearts bring such a spirit—that we can dance like a light being.

Give me massage sessions please. Joints not feeling well. Not liking bits of big home. Being there is very unrestful. My mom is high, brother high, dad low and not on the ground. Im neither here nor there. Again lesson (school) is very exciting and im unable to do it. Its frustrating me so much.

Poems from free writing sessions

Gills of fish bathe in Love
Autism is a fish out of water
All we ask is to be put back into Love
—Sabari

"Happiness"
just blue on the endless sky
winds kindly swaying freer thinking
kind songs for hearts
love never failing
mind full of precious joy
longing never hating
light open hearts
happy hearts awakening
—Sabari

"On Happiness"
very small things give happiness
carefree hearts give happiness
real friends give happiness
dear teachers give happiness
gita bhalla makes a day bright
Vasudha brings freedom
father brings natures gleam
mother very special heart
near and dear bring fun
—Abhishek

"Love and Happiness"
kind moonlight beams
love in the pouring rain
green pointy hills of beauty
pink, caring flowers giving
trees swaying in gratitude
open, lovely loving questions
goodness in thoughts and deeds
reaping hearts open
—Amruth

"A Daisy Dreamer"
Rarest of the daisies dancing
As the quiet, gentle breeze caresses
A golden robed gown
She adorns herself in
And hears the white wind

Hears the hearts sing
Quiet strength she brings
Her food is kind deeds
Hope lives in her seeds
Each day... a gift for her.
—Hari

"Ganga"
O peaceful mother Ganga
I go to you
May your undying waters wash away
Our sins and troubles

Meandering down into fertile lands
Pulling with you luminous light
And hope to feed our lands
With booned particles of rocks

I'm born to die
In your peaceful waters
In Amrit filled luminous waters...

O Mother Ganga
Hear my prayer
Hear me call to you...

> "The White Wind"
> Elegant, verve
> Lungs free
> Beautiful, resplendent fairies
> Singing in choirs
> The Universe hears my song
> Puji just dance. Feels great! Uplifted.
> Joy feels like hundred mountains are being lifted!

Surprising capacities

ASD does not mean mental retardation. In fact the documented prevalence of the "autistic savant" suggests that the opposite is true. Often what is seen is a display of a powerful, but polarized or highly specialized intelligence.

I remember meeting Aditya in Hyderabad—a teenage boy, verbal but diagnosed autistic due to extremely rigid repetitive activities, verbalization and ideas, and prone to violent outbursts. It was extremely difficult for him to read the most obvious social cues. As we walked around his backyard he, quite genuinely, wanted us to enjoy a jasmine bush in flower. Taking a handful of foliage, he repeated "You want to smell it?..smell it?" while literally shoving the flowers and stems up our noses! He also did the same to his own nose.

We saw the sad combination of pure and good intent with a violence and transgression of boundary. Unable to sense the autonomy of the other made his social life impossible, and, as a result, he was confined to his bedroom and hidden from guests and social events.

Yet he could tell you the lowest common denominators of almost any integer in a matter of seconds. Incredible. He had spent his days in his bedroom repeatedly drawing complex geometric shapes studying numbers and mathematics. I sat with Aditya and a calculator. He never paused or made a mistake. I would say 4,688. He would instantly say 1, 2, 4, 8, 16, 293, 586, etc. I would say 56,293. Emotionless, he would say 1, 41, 1,373....

5
An Overview
of Our Approach

"Watch for yourselves and observe the difference—first, when you approach a child more or less indifferently, and then again when you approach him with real love. As soon as you approach him with love, and cease to believe that you can do more with technical fads than you can with love, at once your educating becomes effective, becomes a thing of power. And this is more than ever true when you are having to do with children with special needs..."

—Rudolf Steiner *Curative Education*, lecture 12

How do I see this child with ASD?

In the following drawing, a man is seeing a child in three different ways:

1. As a child who is mentally retarded or deformed in some pathological way

2. As a divine or advanced being—the opposite of the first viewpoint

3. As a child with gifts and hindrances, like all children

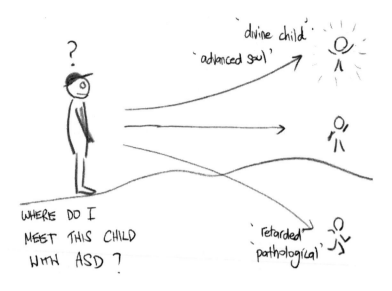

The thing that becomes operational here is the witnessing consciousness of the observer. If we just look at what is happening around the child without preconceived ideas, this could be called phenomenological witnessing. What this means on simple terms is the observer:

- is not seeking to come up with diagnostic labels
- strives to hold an open space, a non-judgmental gaze with warm interest
- cultivates a different way of connection, of communication—not through the usual channels of eye contact and words.

What we can see is that we require a simultaneous perception of all three viewpoints in the diagram.

Overcoming label locked thinking

In her book *The Autistic Brain*, Temple Grandin states that a major limitation among professionals is what she calls "label locked thinking." This is the reductionistic tendency toward diagnosis and treatment plans. It starts with listing deficits and leads to questions such as "what is the single most important thing to do for an autistic child?" or "What do I do to stop a kid who is rocking?" Grandin says herself: "Label locked thinkers want answers. This kind of thinking can do a lot of damage. There is one label—Autism, yet each person does not have the same profile of sensory problems."

She then asks her readers to look to the individual symptoms and sensory profile of each child. Grandin writes about moving from a label to an "actionable diagnosis." When asked about children with special needs, Rudolf Steiner spoke of the need to develop a "useful diagnosis." A useful or actionable diagnosis is not a label, but rather a pointer toward therapy.

Our approach is to peel back the label, slow up the drive toward a solution, and really begin by observation of the fluctuating capacities in different contexts. Also to gather different viewpoints and raise questions relating to the contextual changes in the child's capacity and behaviors.

"Thinking on a symptom by symptom basis will eventually allow us to think about diagnosis and treatment on a patient by patient basis. "
—Temple Grandin, *The Autistic Brain*, p. 115

Here is an example of notes taken during and immediately following the first meeting with one boy:

peripheral gaze; toe walking; rapid frequent hand flapping; no response to his name being called, yet hearing is oversensitive with external sounds—he responds to a motorbike on the street

rigidly held body muscles, shallow breathing, repetitive rocking behaviors; moaning sounds timed with strong rocking movement, restless exploration of the room, briefly touching everything

Response to touch: oversensitive to touch at back of head and neck, yet almost impervious to pain in other parts, e.g., hitting his forehead, scratching his face to the point of blood and scarring

an absence of expressed soul warmth; and people are treated as objects. Yet there are fleeting moments of real eye contact and a sense of connection

These rough notes are not brilliant, clear, objective observations; however, in the sense of a useful or actionable diagnosis they provide indications toward treatment.

The curative education viewpoint

"You will soon realize that there can be no question of expecting simply to be told: This is good for this, and that is good for that. No, what is wanted is a continual living intercourse and connection between your own work and all that is done and given in the educational and in the medical work of the [anthroposophical]

*movement. No break in this living connection
must ever be permitted. Egoism must not be
allowed to creep in and assert itself in some special
and individual activity; rather must there always
be the longing on the part of each participant to
take his right place within the work as a whole."*

The above quote from a lecture course on the topic "curative education" was given in 1924 by Rudolf Steiner in the year before his death. It is clear that Steiner was warning here against "label locked thinking" and generic treatment protocols. He also points toward the need for a group of people to work together, with each one in the right place.

What is interesting is that curative education did not develop as an abstract theory. A small group of young people asked Rudolf Steiner questions about certain children with learning and movement problems. He gathered around him a group of doctors and educators and followed this request up with a period of observation and a series of consultations and discussions. What was new around Rudolf Steiner was the idea of doctors and teachers observing and discussing together. This multiplicity of perspective leading to a flexible, dynamic and ever changing viewpoint informed by different professionals is a central aspect of curative education.

These lectures were given to very small group of pioneers. At the 50th year anniversary of those lectures in 1974, there were over 200 centers around the globe. Since the year 2000 that number has swelled to over 500 centers in more than 40 countries—a truly global movement.

In our work with autism, this curative educational

viewpoint, this co-working, is a core element. There are many obstacles in the structures and legislation of modern educational and medical practices. We are always striving to introduce the idea of shared observation in the study of the child as we have seen time and again how this can bear fruits well beyond what the rational mind would imagine.

In the lecture course, Steiner described these children as *Seelenpflege-bedürftige*—"being in need of special soul care."

What does that mean?

A quote from Carlo Pietzner's booklet *About Curative Education* is helpful here. It also describes beautifully how this "simultaneous perception" may look in practice. Pietzner writes:

> *"The concept implies that by appropriate care and practice the soul-activity of a handicapped person can be guided and stimulated to become a mediator between that individuality and his unwieldy bodily nature. It postulates an intact spiritual entelechy in contrast to a damaged, inadequate or one-sided bodily foundation. But the soul needs help and support if it is to learn to mediate between its higher intention and its imperfect instrument. An element of 'healing' must become active. And that is the foremost ingredient in the 'special soul-care' that Rudolf Steiner provided."*
>
> —Carlo Pietzner, *About Curative Education*

Curative education sees individuality as indestructible. Individuality could also be described as essence, or the spirit—the spiritual individual self beyond the body and soul. Making a connection to an individual's unique essence can lead toward ways of helping. The individual is always more than the challenges he is facing in his body.

Now, after hearing from the children, and having digested the above ideas on the "way of looking" we are ready to summarize key ideas to describe our approach.

FIVE KEY IDEAS

1. Strive to meet the child in their essence (they can sense you doing this)

2. Environmental management rather than behavior management

3. Start with nutrition: support the liver and digestion

4. Next, help them with body image and perception.

5. Build a therapeutic community including parents

1.) Strive to meet the child in their essence

Try to *meet the child* in different contexts—with parents, in the classroom, eating lunch, at home, on the bus, in the playground, during the day and during the night.

Observe how they are with different friends, different family members, and therapists.

Ask: What is constant? What changes with the environment? Observe and document the physical environment, social environment, and sensory environment: color, lighting, sound. How is the child when met with strict expectations?

What about indifference and judgement?

Fear of punishment?

How is the child when met with interest, patience, and love in an unconditionally accepting environment?

Speak with others who know this child. Organise a child study with whoever is willing to do so.

Over time, out of these observations, and from different observers, we build a picture of the essence of the child and begin to get a sense for the quality of their inner life.

Observe and document the life rhythms of the child:

- What do they eat?
- How and when do they eat?
- How and when do they sleep?
- What are their regular bowel habits like and what affects them?

Therapy at the level of life rhythms is crucial. Biorhythms are important internally to organs such as the liver. Lifestyle rhythms connect the human being to the outside world through circadian rhythms (connected to the sun and day/night).

The timing of food and sleep becomes like a medical prescription. Each child requires individualized nutritional content and specific sleep timings. The guiding principle in all of this is:

"*The spirit is intact—the bodily vehicle is unwieldy.*"

This is exactly what the children tell us in their own words as they describe themselves. So we seek through the behaviors to the invisible, to the inner life of the child We do not seek to fix the deficits and excesses. We do not seek to remove, modify, prohibit, punish, or reward.

A helpful idea to meet the essence of the child may be to imagine Beethoven or Mozart playing a solo concert. One would listen to beautiful music emerging from the player and the piano.

Now imagine the same person playing a broken or badly out of tune piano.

What would the music sound like now? And If we had not heard piano music before, what conclusions might we draw about this person's talent or capacity?

2.) Environmental management rather than behavior management

See especially the Introduction; pp. 21–23; and throughout the previous chapters.

3.) Nutrition first

See also the appendix on nutrition.

There is a pattern in medicine and epidemiology that, for many so-called behavioral problems, causation is first considered to be psychological, then gradually the brain and neurons seem to be the culprits, and finally attention descends to the lower part of the human being, the metabolism and digestion.

Largely because of the prevalence of autism and ADHD, there has been growing evidence regarding the connection between the gut and the brain. This information is becoming more mainstream now. The Australian Autism & ADHD Foundation, for example, cites research suggesting that "these disorders are associated with genetic predispositions triggered by environmental factors…such as a "Western style" diet, consisting of too many nutrient-poor refined foods, additives, preservatives and colorings, and other chemicals."

4.) Feeling the body: proprioception and body perception

I can't feel the ends of my hands and I am unaware of pressure. —Sabari

Eric Chen, a Chinese boy we met in Singapore wrote this about his relationship to his body:

The Autistic boy
Who had a body that was never right
a body that never tells him what it is feeling
a body that never listened to his will
like being stuck in an alien submarine,
in the depths of the ocean.

If we take direction from the words of the children, we find striking descriptions of a child who has a body, who has limbs, yet cannot feel them. One must really take a moment to imagine what that would be like.

Proprioception is the ability to feel and adapt one's own muscle contractions and also to feel, adjust to and balance the effects of gravity. Research involving astronauts has revealed that time spent away from the forces of gravity leads to a condition of reading words in a jumbled way—backwards and upside down—its caused by zero gravity environment and is called "space dyslexia."

The children report the feeling of being disconnected from their bodies; they report a sense of witnessing themselves, rather than inhabiting their bodily flesh.

One of the most fascinating aspects of Temple Grandin's journey (as shown in the film about her life)

is her "squeeze machine." She developed a large wooden box where she could crawl in on hands and knees, pull a lever to experience being squeezed strongly by the movable wooden walls. This would calm her down during moments of uncontrollable anxiety, preventing public meltdowns. We can understand this from the perspective of body perception and proprioception. The squeeze machine gives a powerful experience of the location of the body in space.

Body perception can be helped by massage and often by firm touch. Rhythmical massage and craniosacral are highly refined and sensitive forms of body oriented therapies. Hand gesture games can be highly therapeutic. Other movement therapies involving structured rhythmic movement address the bodily senses in different ways include curative eurythmy, morning circle activities in class, dance, gymnastics, and team sports.

From a sensory-psychological perspective, an inability to feel ones own body movement has a profound effect on baseline feelings of being grounded, calm, and safe. Higher functions such as communication and socialization require the feeling of oneself as a center of consciousness. Rudolf Steiner's groundbreaking work on the twelve senses gives a framework to understand this.

Work with proprioception (the sense of movement), and the vestibular system (the sense of balance) is essential in autism treatment. These need to be individualized for each child with different sensory processing challenges. Activities can take the form of simple touch and massage techniques practiced by parents and caregivers. There is also a wide range of age appropriate children's games, including hand gesture games accompanied by speech and song. Classroom activities and curriculum can be developed with sensory processing in mind—this is what we did in the schools where we worked. Curative education curriculum is based on a deep knowledge of the interconnection of the twelve senses, in particular the idea that speech formation requires and emerges from a well developed sense of movement. This is an extensive topic and can only be touched upon in this book.

5.) Autism calls for a healing community including parents and family

Therapy for autism requires a community of people: doctors, teachers, therapists, parents and family. The child receives something from each individual, but what is more is what the child receives from being surrounded by the warm relationships developed in the healing community.

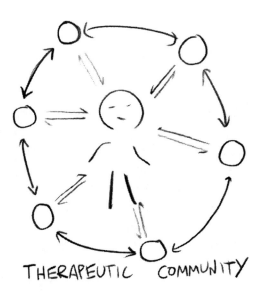

THERAPEUTIC COMMUNITY

These people should come together regularly to review progress, modify programs, and hear from others about their different perspectives on the child. This helps the *total picture* of the child to emerge, not just fragments of the whole. Particularly in the treatment of autism, the child may be attending therapies all over town—occupational therapy, speech therapy, ABA, massages, horseback riding, music therapy, etc. Often, all these things are delivered to the child in bits and fragments. The child with autism lacks this power of integration. There is lack of integrative forces from inside the child, so the therapeutic principle is to bring integration from the outside. This can be done in the social realm.

Leading the process may be a doctor, a teacher, or a parent. The real leader is the essence of the child; however, this essence operates from behind a veil. We have found that children respond positively when this circle is functioning well. The therapeutic circle is a self-organizing group of people. It works when everyone has the highest interest of the child held in their hearts. This communal will can create a self-managing, service-oriented, and dynamic structure.

The challenge is to create a spiritually aware therapeutic community. There will be many different people in the life of a child on the spectrum. Can each person find their place with their specific contribution, and also recognize what others bring to the whole circle around the child?

Each person in the child's life brings their individual gifts, but in the service of one child. This is the way we have built therapeutic communities. We have tried to do this in South India in the various centers because we found that the more services are delivered as a whole—integrated and held in a network of warmth and shared interest—the better the children respond.

As we can see in the picture of the therapeutic circle around the child, more important than the type of therapy is the *relationships between therapists, teachers, and parents.*

This expanded model of sensory integration requires that the child is held in an integrated and cohesive social web of helpers. The role of the physician is to oversee this multi-disciplinary integrative landscape of therapists and educators. It requires time for meeting in person and training in a commonly held image of the child.

6

THERAPY DIRECTIONS: CONCLUSIONS AND BEGINNINGS

"The uppermost requirement of therapy for an autistic is love and firmness; the therapy is useless without love, because love triggers a resounding response internally. The autistic is forlorn and lonely. The autistic fully appreciates love, but is hampered very much by lack of communication."
—Krishna Narayan, *Wasted Talent: Musings of an Autistic*

"Any therapeutic intervention must help the child in the direction of motivated or intentional action. This is the only way that a human being is able to influence its future destiny."
—Rudolf Steiner, *Curative Education*

What are the steps toward a useful educational approach and helpful therapies? How do we prepare ourselves to be able to hear Prasaad's call to *meet me who I am*? Our mindset and practice can be informed by the five key points from the previous chapter.

- Strive to meet the child in their essence

- Environmental management rather than behavior management

- Nutrition
- Body image and perception
- Build a therapeutic community including the parents

Now we add more practical examples and concluding thoughts.

Curriculum

One indication that seemed to help the Indian children was to spend long periods of time on the same theme. The Steiner/Waldorf curriculum is structured in content blocks of three to four weeks. At Saandeepani and V-Excel we stayed on the same topics for three to six months. This allowed for repeated and prolonged artistic exploration around a theme, for example, Ancient Greece—including music, drawing, painting, movement, and drama. We found that children could really live into and take in the content through this repeated and prolonged artistic presentation. Barely verbal children began to sing, and paintings and drawings were produced. The children became more active in their limbs; more alive in their will.

The aim of this method of content delivery is not the regurgitation of learned material. It is a medium to connect with children at the level of feeling and soul. As teachers found at V-Excel: "Then, after the lessons in Ancient Greek and Norse myth there was a shift—suddenly there was more communication. And the communication became more clear, more coherent."

Prasaad describes a change in his capacity to execute his conscious intention through his limbs here:

I find an inner change in me here.

I am not in charge of myself only with my stomach.

My great sun like head bears a thought which I can put into action.

I go not with a feeling but a thought.

I think my own thought from within me—my intention.

It is mine, mine to feel.

I had a thought to paint something, and I could actually do it.

If I wanted to paint Hector and Achilles I could.

It brought me great joy.

Unless I get this gift of thought into action, I cant be independent.

ASD feels liberated during these sessions.

Social integration

Take every opportunity for integration into real life: shopping, parks, libraries, swimming, festivals. With the experience of something new, behavioral fixations and stimming can increase and overpower the child temporarily. Remember that behind rigid, repetitive behaviors, or fixation of thoughts, there is the gesture of self-protection. Or one could say the gesture of self-realization—the struggle to feel secure in oneself; to identify with oneself. Sometimes escalations of these behaviors can be extremely troubling, especially when they occur in public, so when working with individual children in specific areas of rigidity or fixations, it is helpful to carry an understanding of social integration.

Some helpful questions to ask when dealing with fixations:

- Why is their a need for the object of the fixation?
- How does the object of fixation provide protection?
- What is the inner sensory process that is active here?
- How can I allow this need in an appropriate way?

Think of a two-year-old throwing a tantrum, to the point that they are, in a way, "stuck" in that state—they themselves can't get out of it. Often a verbal command does not get through at all—but perhaps the offer of a snack, or a glass of water, or a sincere hug will settle the behavior.

Who can sense this and act on it? How do we sense what a child needs?

Only in the space of love can I sense this, when looking without judgement and with warm interest. The child senses that you sense them, then, whatever you do will work. That is the real key to therapy.

Dr. Karl König, the early pioneer in curative education expressed the same idea in this way:

> "Only the help from human to human—the en-
> counter of "I" with another "I"... the becoming
> aware of the other person's individuality... simply
> the meeting, eye to eye, of two persons creates that
> curative education which counters, in a healing way,
> the threat to our inmost humanity. This can only
> be effective if with it a fundamental recognition
> happens—a recognition which has to come out of
> the heart."

There will be many different people in the life of a child on the spectrum. We have asked this question: Can each person find their place with their specific contribution and also recognize what others bring in the whole circle around each child?

Our experience has shown us that this *is possible*; and that when it happens you are likely to see the marvelous leaps, gains, and progress that lie dormant in the realm of our hopes and dreams for these children. Reading accounts of children who have moved off the spectrum or "recovered," you often find that, in fact, it is the people around the child who have undergone a complete transformation. When that happens, the child can walk along the "bridge of warmth" created by the love, learning, and efforts of the community. Then they walk, speak and find themselves able to be amongst us, in a circle they have themselves collected, transformed, and humanized. Prasaad uses the metaphor of the "key to unlocking" this bridge of warmth, and directs us to our own hearts, our inner life:

> *They (teachers) are the key and the doorway to unlocking this great amount of responsibility on their shoulders and their hearts in looking inwards and changing themselves.*

The bridge of human warmth

American pediatrician Michael Allen, who himself raised a child with special needs said in an interview with *Lilipoh* magazine:

> *"People who are handicapped bring in karmic blessings and karmic work for parents, siblings, caregivers—anyone and everyone who has a relationship with them in any way. This is a real Christ healing impulse to learn social connection,*

and how to care for our fellow human beings. Each handicap brings a specific lesson for the individual, parents, family and community."

Recent developments in Western medicine, at least in theory, have also moved in this direction of acknowledging the social, psychological and spiritual dimension of illness since the 1970s as evidenced by the Primary Health Care movement. This approach emphasizes:

- the social determinants of health as against a narrow biomedical view of causation

- a focus on environmental medicine, illnesss prevention and population health

- community participation and involvement in health

- a multi-sectorial approach—e.g., linking health and education sectors

Even that far back, leading lights of the World Health Organization began to speak of a "bio-psycho-social" approach, and of an outlook that seeks to examine both health and illness in a way which is meaningful in the life of an individual human being. In recent years especially with relation to work in indigenous communities with inherent spiritual beliefs the catch phrase often heard at conferences and in published papers has become "a bio-psycho-social-spiritual approach."

The disappointing thing to see is how much these ideals of the global WHO remain in the conceptual realm in the practice of health care. In relation to autism research, ways of thinking and understanding the world over are heavily biased towards biomedical causality and chemical excess/deficit based treatments. In many cases thinking is chained to the biomedical model. What does this do? It chains us all to pharmaceuticals as our only hope and answer. Medical research and development scan, test and sample on the level of the physical body, seeking chemical imbalances and drugs to fix it. In the case of autism/ADHD these drugs are psychoactive—Increasingly we have the situation that it's normal to dose young children with psychoactive drugs: Ritalin is a case in point.

One striking piece of evidence connects Ritalin with elevated "accident proneness" and an elevated frequency of accidents. A large scale German study found that serious injuries in children were associated with Ritalin use at a frequency rate of 6 times more than the control group. Children have accidents more often when they are disconnected from their bodily senses, their somatic nature. (See Grützmacher H, "Unfallgefährdung bei Aufmerksamkeits und Hyperaktivitätsstörung," *Deutsches Ärzteblatt* Jg. 98 Heft 34-35 27. Aug. 2001.)

In addition to this, the so called "alternative" medical movement in recent years is beginning to look more and more like a caricature of the biomedical model. How many organizations and websites are blaming lack or excess of certain minerals and then selling them?

This impasse leads us precisely to the domain of curative education and anthroposophic medicine.

"Anthroposophic medicine is a holistic and human-centered approach to medicine. It is practiced by physicians who have done a conventional medical training, but expand conventional scientific views by incorporating an understanding of the laws of the living organism, and the emotional and spiritual aspects of the human being. Instead of trying to define illness into particular categories

*and to standardize treatment for a given disease,
anthroposophic medicine strives to recognize the
unique aspects of an individual person's constitution
and biographical path."* —Dr. Adam Blanning

A practitioner of anthroposophic medicine seeks to place illness in not a narrow, but the widest possible context. A teacher trained in curative education becomes a scientist of relationship. A true soul-spiritual approach extends this even further. It asks the question why is autism increasing at such an alarming rate in modern civilized society? What could it mean? What is being asked of us?

In his interview, Dr. Allen goes on to describe the dramatic increase of autism as a phenomenon well beyond the domain of individual genetics, family history, birth trauma, environmental toxins and vaccines. It is a perspective which encompasses contextually the whole of Western civilization and the rapid industrial/technological/economic growth of recent history. The result of this rapid change is that the inside of each and every home, the daily life of children looks so very different to what it did even twenty years ago.

*"According to educator Eugene Schwartz, if we
look at illnesses as mirrors for the age, we see in
our current mirror, indifference, social isolation,
timidity, and lack of empathy. In autism we find
individuals who share these characteristics and
serve as sacrificial mirrors to reflect our time.*

*"Ours is a time of materialism. This excessive ma-
terialism distracts us from our spiritual development. This is a sign of our times. The purpose of
autism is to balance out this excessive materialism.*

Thus autism can be seen as both the result of, and the remedy for, excessive materialism. We are suffering from the inability to develop spiritually and deeply connect with our fellow human beings. Autism reveals this to us, and gives us the opportunity to step away from ourselves and our immersion in the materialistic world, and focus on helping our children with autism and the world at large. We have to be sensitive, caring, and loving enough to open ourselves to the gifts that these individuals bring to the world. With healthy empathy and tolerance, we can support them and learn the meaning and balance of their incarnation. In the process, we learn to strive for healthy social connection and continue developing our potential as spiritual human being."

—Michael Allen, MD, FAAP, ABIHM, ACAM

What we have observed over and over is parents of autistic children disillusioned, upset even angered by a failing medical system and the lack of empathy and understanding they have received. Ultimately, this pushes parents to become researchers—reading and exploring everything in the search to understand and help. They themselves are becoming evidence-based researchers—observing directly their child and then sharing online the effects of a course of speech therapy, chelation, or a trial of nutritional changes. The internet is flooded with this information with parents, professionals and families navigating the conflicting streams of thought.

Rudolf Steiner did say that at around the time of the new millennium there will be so much conflicting information on offer in the scientific world that one will not know the difference between right and wrong. That turned out to be a prophetic warning. He goes on to say that precisely this dilemma will provide a great opportunity for the individualization process that he spent his life describing. Illness can be seen in the context of this individualization process, as the battle of the individual soul against the dehumanising nature forces in the environment. Writing about curative education, sir Laurens Van Der Post critiques the "industrialization of the West, the rationalization of the European spirit, growing materialism and the severance of man from his instinctive self" and in his view Rudolf Steiner's work "stands and remains alive, relevant and dynamic." Curative education brings "balance and compensation to the deprivation and disproportion of this century which Steiner's spirit so imaginatively confronted."

The remedy is not an easy pill, and, like autism, it is multi-dimensional, heavily dependent on relationship. In our times, it is not only the child with autism who requires both wisdom and love to find and express their essence and their gifts. This is our challenge as a global community of parents and educators.

This book, inspired by the children we have met, encourages the reader to take a broad contextual view of the child with autism. Our years of work with individual children has led us to this broader "whole systems" view of each child in his or her complex changing environmental context. The environment also includes people and the quality of human relationships around the child.

Carl Jung described the human journey from birth towards individuation. In his early writings he describes the polarity between individuation and its opposite—what he calls "Abraxas." Abraxas is the sum total of all the impersonal forces acting on the human being—all the forces of nature: gravity, chemistry, physics—the great cycles of creation and destruction. These forces are also expressed in the Hindu trinity of Creation (Brahma), Preservation (Vishnu), and Destruction/Renewal (Shiva).

Each human soul is placed in a body and lives in the midst of Abraxas. Rudolf Steiner names individualization as the goal of human evolution. Steiner, however, highlights one more twist to the story—individualization, at a certain point, becomes dependent on community. In terms of development and evolution, Steiner's work places great emphasis on the meeting, the encounter, between two or more human beings. This idea informs his practical advice on education and medicine.

When we look at the increasing phenomenon of autism in modern times with these contextual thoughts in mind, we just might be able to move from being lost within the "autism puzzle" toward seeing the whole and some meaningful directions.

Taking a historic, evolutionary perspective, we have seen a rapid industrialization in the last few hundred years. Many cultures on the globe are trying to integrate a scientific worldview with more traditional spiritually-oriented cultures. In our experience, ASD is more common in urban industrialized areas. Is the rise in autism reflecting this global change?

If we take a whole systems view, one could say the whole world has become one-sided—oriented to materialism. For many modern illnesses we are beginning to find causation in the combined effects of pollutants, environmental toxins, vaccines, and modern food and farming methods.

However, in general, we can say that autism is inability to handle matter.

From the ingestion of food to the handling of objects like pens, the child with autism struggles to make use of the things of this earth, of matter. As a general rule they do not move on to successful careers and high paying jobs in the economic system. The much higher prevalence among boys (four to one, male vs. female) is interesting in this light.

But they do point us toward a sober reassessment of so many aspects of modern life. In particular, parenting and child rearing. They point us toward deepening our relationships—they bring a spirituality—an orientation to non-material aspects of existence. If behavior is language, then the child with autism may be speaking something like this:

> *"I need help to individualize. I am oversensitive, overly subject to the external world, therefore, my behavior will reflect my environment. I magnify what lives in the environment and make it visible. Please don't punish me for that but seek to understand me. I want to change. I can change more easily if there is a change in my environment. You, dear friend are part of my environment."*

We of the dominant culture try to fix them. Holding tight to our perspective and professionalism we colonize them, and try to change their worldview toward our own "neuro-typical" experience. We categorize them and even socially isolate them. And then we try to keep living our lives in the same way as we did before. How will it look if this tendency to classify, diagnose, segregate, and treat "abnormal behavior" continues unchecked?

"Essentially we do not really have the right to talk about normality or abnormality in a child's inner life, nor indeed in the inner life of human beings altogether... One does not gain much from such labelling, and the first thing to happen should be that the physician or the teacher rejects such an assessment."—Rudolf Steiner

We can find answers by living with those living with
autism.

By building communities where we share life and
hold interest in each other.

We don't force them to become us.

We don't want to become them.

Then we begin to see thru their eyes, to experience
thru their sensory profile.

Then from this effort, parallel journeys can begin.

They enter our world.

They start to see the world through our eyes.

We develop a compassion for their efforts, their
struggles.

We learn to understand behaviors as script and
language.

Windows begin to open.

Communication requires this warm space.

"Behavior change" flows naturally on from this.

The work is actually this:

How do we develop the faculties of understanding the
other?

Not through silent spiritual exercises and
meditation, but through practical work with these
children,
Through striving to sense their invisible needs.
Then an alchemy happens.
The therapeutic community around the child—
family, therapists, doctors, teachers—
We all build relationships—warm relationships—
that the children can imitate .
We become worthy of their imitation.
There comes a day when we build a new culture.
It's no longer so one-sided, with materialistic values.
It's more balanced and humanized.
This is the future human culture.
It emerges from a real and true engagement with
autistic people.
When we receive what they are bringing to us.
They come with heightened faculties into a world
that is not able to recognize these faculties
Or make them useful.
So they appear strange to us.
These faculties become pathological—
hypersensitivity becomes not coping.
For a musician, sensitivity to sound becomes a
career.
For Temple Grandin, sensitivity to animals became a
vocation.
The writings of our children in Chennai are powerful
works.

They can change us.

If we recognize the gift each child brings: hold their hand, help them to overcome hinderances

Then, together, we relocate what was a disability,

Into a movement for development and transformation.

This is the message of the children with whom we have journeyed.

That is what a gang of non-verbal adolescent boys called "free hearts,

Have named as their covert mission: "Operation Love."

A mystery and a burden transforms into wings and flight.

Final words: From the inner life

Two of our children wrote (actually only one of them wrote, but he said it was the thoughts of his friend):

ON FREEDOM

Inside me
Infinite birds
Live in families of caged dreams.

I seek the key
I seek the lock which I build

Outside me there lies no cage
Within me there lies the key.

Where do I entrap myself?
Why do I feel locked in?
Freedom is lived
Not given or taken.

This is my simple message today.

Free yourself from blame, from hurt, from pain.
Because only you can.

—Amruth and Shiva

Appendix

Nutrition, Restricted Diet, and Reintegration of Foods

There are many layers to be aware of when working with children on the spectrum in the area of nutrition. To start with, there are different ways of understanding the word nourishment—i.e., physically through food, through the senses, and also through warm trusting relationships. As some children grew up and started expressing through art and poetry, that also was a different kind of nourishment, more in the realm of the soul.

But here I want to share about my experiences and insights around working with food rhythms, choosing foods to eat in individual children at different stages of healing work and the outcomes of these practices.

Even though I am writing from the perspective of the specific diet a child is on or not on, I want to emphasize that children are experiencing a variety of sensory and relational aspects simultaneously. So in reality, it is hard to separate all these intricately connected factors working on these children in the same time and space. Diet programs happen in relation to rest of the life experiences mentioned and the changing sensory world of that child, sleep habits, and the immediate important relationships around that child.

This understanding takes us away from focusing on actual dietary restrictions and allowances at the physical level and takes us on a journey into the child's inner life through these changing life rhythms. So I am asking the focus to be shifted from objectively measurable physical diet programs to keen observation of the actual process of moving in and out of different food protocols. Observation of what? Where to direct our focus? To the child's inner experience.

The primary question then becomes: How is the child on this or that diet showing or expressing their inner experience? Learning to understand how the child is experiencing their inner life and studying it with sensitivity was my first step toward working with lifestyle rhythms.

In my work with these children, I sat with the family and we mutually agreed upon a twelve-week program of dietary restrictions. Many times in practice, especially in the early years of my work, this was not easy. It is asking parents to move into a totally new way of feeding their child. This in many instances was simply not possible for parents who were already living under enormous amount of stress. Some parents never slept even one whole night peacefully.

But now after many years of seeing the effects of diet change in hundreds of cases and an established and proven work, the team knew what positive changes to expect out of this challenging step. We entered this with anticipation of this positive outcome as a powerful incentive.

What do we do as first step? We go into detail of the delivery of three main meals and established rhythms of day and night.

At a glance, this is how it looks:

Breakfast: before 9 am; gluten free grain & protein (heaviest meal)

Lunch: between noon and 1 pm; gluten free grain & protein with vegetables

Dinner: between 5:30 and 7 pm; gluten free grain & protein with vegetable (easily digested /lightest meal)

No grain or protein at any time other than main meal times.

Some foods were totally eliminated on this program:

- All gluten-containing grains
- Milk and milk products except clarified butter (ghee)
- All processed, preserved and refined foods
- All fruits
- Some vegetables are given with limited frequency

This strict elimination brought us to a very simple, consistent program.

My original work, in early years was with south Indian families. I had enormous challenges removing milk and milk products—yoghurt and milk are culturally important in South India. I met the disapproving stares of many traditional grandmothers wondering what on earth I was talking about!

On the other hand, some of the old traditional recipes from these parts of world served our program well. In urbanized India, shops and local stores had become full of processed, packaged food by this stage. Essentially most families needed to go back to their old traditional way of cooking for children, except without milk and yoghurt.

In the later part of my research, I learned that many old traditional tribal communities from Andhra Pradesh state actually feed their children in a similar way to our program and in these remote communities, until today, elders do not report knowledge of such a thing as autism.

Once I established this simple, rhythmic, consistent way of nourishing children with warm, home cooked, locally grown grains and proteins, I entered the next layer of work.

Working with detox / supplementation

Working with and integrating the fruits of many peoples work over the last 50 years around gut-brain syndrome was my first natural step as a trained pediatrician. The book *Children with Starving Brains* was published at around the same time as I met my first batch of children, the early years before Saandeepani. The author, Dr. J McCandless, being both a medical doctor and parent of a child on the spectrum, explored deeply the gut-brain connection and also the biomedical approach.

Children in Saandeepani on these established rhythmic, restricted diets began taking locally acting antifungal medication and probiotic supplementation. Some children also began taking zinc\copper supplementations.

We had children who entered our program with already established supplementation programs started by other practitioners from around the world. Indian parents reached out far and wide for help. We did not disturb these protocols and programs in these children, but included them into our stream. This resulted in me having to experience children who were on many different diet supplementation programs in the same group.

Even though there was a definite understanding of what we were doing and where we were going in this program with gut strengthening, there was openness and variation created by each individual child's needs and circumstances.

Parents had so many questions and began speaking of *"freedom within the boundary."* There was structure (and rules) around eating and sleeping, but within that every individual family need was accommodated.

During this early period of research, I came across *Wasted Talent,* a book by Krishna Narayanan. I followed up on his suggestion that more research is needed into Ayurvedic work, because it helped his recovery from autism. That took me on a journey to Kerala State and into learning from traditional Ayurvedic healers.

My unique personal journey here involves integrating three separate paths:
1. my biochemical understanding from mainstream medical research on the gut and brain
2. Ayurvedic medical wisdom
3. Lectures and writings from Rudolf Steiner and Dr. Ita Wegman—the inner path of anthroposophy

This inner contemplative, scientific path guided by anthroposophy took me into a process of living with children on the spectrum to build physical diagnostic pictures. From those objective phenomenological observations, the challenge to then bring up meditative pictures for contemplation resulted in the beginning of spiritual research into autism.

Interestingly, this is also the essence of autism for me: To work on the level of the physical, but working with this level through spiritual pictures behind every physical manifestation. I worked in this way with every child.

Within this framework of restricted, rhythmic ways of nourishing, what specific, individual aspects are crucial for each set of parents? What questions do I need ask in order to understand why following the diet is difficult for this or that child's family? These questions led me beyond the scope of what is usually done in the consultation room. On one occasion, it was helping to build the relation between grandmother and parents who lived together with the child —bridging a gap between them. Both the parents and grandmother needed to work together to bring this food program into practice.

For another child, the mother needed to find friends in our community to help her with recipes. And in other, the mother needed to get the whole family on this program, and then witnessed the entire family benefiting. And so on, and on….

What I am trying to convey here is, even though the diet program is simple, it is the journey of each family around that child which became central to me. Accompanying every family in this journey with different pathways, sensing and meeting the needs that were arising out of each specific situation brought me to a point of new understanding.

In the cases where the entire family moved into a new life style and new way of relating to each other and to the external world, the need for further steps into detox programs or supplementation became less and less. And where need was felt because of the parent's concerns, it was addressed through food. Some *helpful factors in detoxing* follow.

Liver rhythms

Food timings and sleep rhythms support healthy liver function. The liver is the body's detoxification center.

Using Black Millet [Ragi]: This helps in both detox and mineral supplementation. Ragi is offered as a drink or as cooked grain as part of the main meal.

Supporting the family in allowing natural detox reactions to occur in children without suppressing them (for example, rashes, cold and cough reactions, behavioral changes).

Where needed, children were given natural, remedies to support digestive and liver processes.

As far as possible, mineral supplementations were provided through food. Where required, natural supplements were chosen, e.g., the various anthroposophic preparations of Iron.

In all cases, I engaged the family in many dialogues about the child's daily routine. This conscious engagement with parents and grandparents around daily life rhythms had positive influences on children's outcome. Some of the changes we observed with children who followed these protocols are improvement in sleep and better cognitive processing, and these changes usually started becoming obvious after a period of twelve weeks.

The longer the child is on consistent programs, the better and more sustainable positive changes are established. In older children, sometimes it took six to twelve months before we could observe some changes. Areas where we documented positive outcomes are attention span and social behaviors. These children always responded better to any kind of sensory therapies, and positive response to therapy was always more consistent and sustainable in children on diet programs.

Some families needed more support and over longer periods to come into this new life style and to maintain it without breaks. In some situations whole communities of teachers, therapists, and school management needed to participate in parent support.

Reintroduction of foods (the beginning of sensing the self through the body)

Roughly at this stage where everyday life has become more easily manageable, discussions about reintroduction started. Of course, as with everything else, it was very different from family to family. Some parents did not even want to talk about looking back; they were very comfortable and needing to move forward without any changes.

But with some families, we entered this discussion as soon as parents felt relaxed about managing everyday routines, such as eating, sleeping, etc. In my work, I noticed that constipation took a much longer time than some other symptoms to respond.

Typically, we introduced one new item at a time—roughly once a week—watching closely for any symptoms. These children responded with hyperactivity or disturbed sleep for every change initially. If we continued with the new change, symptoms improved over one or two weeks. Foods that were chosen in the reintroduction plan were fruits with less sugar content and, for some children, dairy products.

I want to share some of my observations during reintroduction.

Most of the children could express or become aware of pain in the tummy with new food, which was not present a few months before. Some even rejected the food, saying "it hurts."

This waking up to their own inner life was the beginning of something new. Where we observed this certain new faculty of self-consciousness, progress and development followed.

This deep relation between *how one senses ones own inner life* and cognitive reception as well as comprehension and expressive communication skills has become one of the key factors in working with these children.

This is where I learned my next big step, moving on from working with nutrition to enter a pathway into supporting each child's soul needs.

Changes in diet programs resulted in something waking up in the child deep inside, a waking up to perception of the self. What then followed was a noticeable change in perception of the world and other people. This manifested as increased attention span, increased eye contact, better comprehension of instructions, and a certain calmness in demeanor.

Many children never reached optimum health in their gut and needed to remain vigilant with certain foods. But, through taking this journey of restrictive diet and then the reintroduction of certain foods definitely changed almost every child in this aspect of "sensing the self."

The previously required behavior management and external regulation was replaced with something coming naturally from within the child. We began to see, for the first time, self-restraint, planning, and more moments of engagement and participation. In some children, we saw a dramatic leap of change, including the emergence of speech. Some children moved into more academic settings.

I would like to close this for the time being, this chapter on nutritional programs for autism, with a quote from Rudolf Steiner, which best describes where we are at this time with this work.

> *Healing and Education — and the two are, as you know, nearly related—do not depend so much on concocting all kinds of mixtures — be they physical or psychical!—but on knowing exactly what can really help.*
>
> —Rudolf Steiner, *Curative Education*, lecture five

The field of autism is where I have experienced this concoction of all kinds of thoughts, opinions, and belief systems. I know some children who take over 50 supplements daily. Some families are running between five and ten different therapies weekly. Often parents gather and work with the opinions of many doctors and specialists, each with their own protocols. And yet, every child is asking us to meet him or her at a very individual point.

I sometimes wonder whether the pathway to know exactly what helps is to go through these concoctions of all kinds of mixtures.

This picture also reminds me how our human metabolic system deals with all the substances from outside world and miraculously manages to work with individual specific wisdom in its protein synthesis. Steiner continues:

What is important then, is to be able to know in any particular case what particular substance is required; we must really succeed in following the path that brings us to that knowledge.
—Rudolf Steiner, *Curative Education*, lecture five

Meeting every child on the spectrum, with the above question as physician, took me on a circuitous, rich, rewarding, and fruitful journey. I had to ask *what is the specific substance or therapy or required change for this child at this moment?* This is one place where my spiritual practice and meditative path became helpful in finding answers. I was learning to bring up, out of the physical experience of observing the child, meditative pictures. And every time, with every child, a new journey, a new meeting.

About the Authors

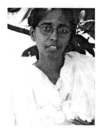Dr. Lakshmi Prasanna is a pediatrician with a specialty in neonatology and a special interest in autism. She directed a neonatal intensive care unit for 15 years and now runs a curative center for special needs children in Hyderabad, South India. Co-founder and president of the Anthroposophical Medical Society in India, she has worked extensively in India and Australia as a lecturer and health educator, particularly within school communities.

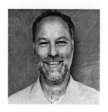Michael Kokinos is a physiotherapist with a clinical practice in Australia, Blue Sky Therapies, specializing in craniosacral work. He has worked extensively on innovative health care projects with government and Aboriginal leaders in the remote North of Australia, and visits India regularly, mainly to support families of autistic children and conduct joint workshops with Dr. Lakshmi Prasanna for therapists, special educators and parents.

CPSIA information can be obtained
at www.ICGtesting.com
Printed in the USA
FFOW04n1447250118
44731372-44773FF